The NEW
Psoa[s] [Relea]se Party!

Rele[ase]
Chronic Pain and [B...]

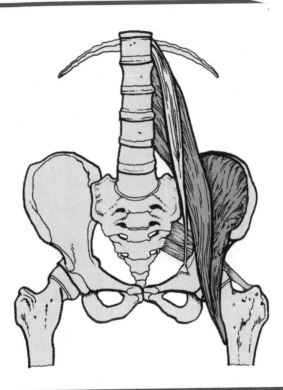

by Jonathan FitzGordon

Other books in this series:

Sciatica/Piriformis Syndrome
The Spine: An Introduction To The Central Channel
The Exercises of CoreWalking
CoreWalking: First Steps to A New Yourself

Cover Illustation: Frank Morris

TABLE OF CONTENTS

I The Wonder Muscle 1

II The Psoas in Infancy 13

III The Psoas Is a Pulley....................................21

IV Muscles That Support the Psoas 31

V The Effects of a Tight Psoas........................47

VI The Psoas and the Organs 53

VII The Psoas and the Nervous System..........59

VIII Releases..67

IX Stretches...89

X Psoas Blog Posts..99

Acknowledgements..257

FOUR VIEWS OF THE PSOAS MUSCLE

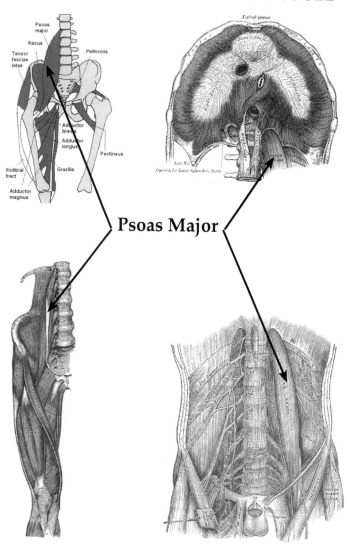

Psoas Major

Chapter I

THE WONDER MUSCLE

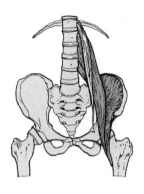

As a yoga teacher, I was taught to stretch people, but it wasn't long before I began to come across people who didn't seem to be served by stretching. They would come to class with dogged regularity, but their hips or hamstrings or whatever they hoped to lengthen never seemed to acquiesce. I came to realize that a muscle that is full of tension cannot be stretched free of that tension. In certain cases we must learn to release the tension and/or trauma from a muscle in order to get to the point where we can stretch it.

Deep in the bowl of the pelvis lies the psoas major, the body's most important muscle, which many people have never heard of. This muscle, my favorite, is both the main engine of movement and the main recipient/warehouse for trauma.

The human body is a miraculous creation, an intricately designed machine in which every part plays a specific role in trying to keep the body in a state of balance. It is a balance that crosses many spectrums—muscular, skeletal, emotional, physiological, etc.—and this elusive balance requires a great deal of harmony among disparate parts of the body.

THE PSOAS MAJOR

At the center of it all is the iliopsoas muscle group, three muscles lining the core of the body on either side. The psoas major is the body's main hip flexor and one of only three muscles connecting the lower and upper body. When healthy, the psoas major in front and the piriformis (gluteus maximus is the third muscle) across the back help us stand upright in a perfect state of balance. The psoas attaches along the lower spine and comes down to cross over the rim of the pelvis before it moves backward again to insert on the back half of the inner thigh. The tension that the psoas creates across the rim of the pelvis as it moves backward at its top and bottom is critical to healthy upright posture.

The second muscle of the iliopsoas is the iliacus, which has a similar job to the psoas. The iliacus muscle lines the bowl of the pelvis and meets the psoas major to form a common tendon that inserts on the back half of the inner thigh.

The third muscle of the iliopsoas muscle group is a very interesting muscle called the psoas minor. It is considered to be a devolving muscle—according to anatomy books, only 50 percent of the population has this muscle.

The psoas major connects at six points—it attaches at the base of the rib cage and the top of the lower back. It connects to the outer edge of the first four vertebrae of the lumbar spine, which is the lower back, and to the front of these vertebrae as well as the front of the 12th thoracic vertebra, which is at the base of the rib cage, and it crosses over the front of the pelvis and goes backward to attach on the back half of the inner thigh, on a bony projection called the lesser trochanter. As a result the psoas spans and affects many joints.

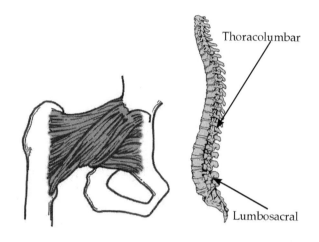

Thoracolumbar

Lumbosacral

There are many important joints or junctures in the body, but I always return to four particular ones that involve the psoas. These are the two femoral joints, where each leg meets the hip bones of the pelvis; the lumbosacral, where the pelvis meets the spine; and the thoracolumbar, where the lower (lumbar) and middle back (thoracic) meet. This last spot is where I see the most fundamental postural collapse in most of my clients. Improper alignment of the skeletal system always leads to imbalances in the muscular system, and vice versa.

The placement of the pelvis determines a great deal of what happens in the legs, trunk and arms. Again, the psoas is one of only three muscles that connect the upper and lower body, and even though it doesn't connect to the

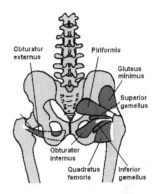

pelvis (57 other muscles do), it exerts a profound influence over its alignment. The other two muscles are the piriformis, which attaches the leg to the sacrum and the psoas connects the body across the front and the piriformis at the back. These two muscles, when working well(along with gluteus maximus), perform a balancing act that allows for successful upright posture. A problem with one of these muscles always involves a problem with the other, as well.

When the psoas is in an unhappy state, there are a host of physical conditions that can be connected to its issues—lower-back pain, hip pain, groin pain, bladder problems, constipation, poor circulation, leg-length discrepancy, scoliosis, bad menstrual cramps, and the list goes on and on. For instance, a chronically tight psoas on both sides pulls the vertebrae of the lower back forward, which can lead to pain due to compression of the joints and discs of the lower spine. If the psoas is tight on just one side, it can trigger a contraction of that entire side, causing one leg to be shorter than the other; it may even lead to the curvature of the spine known as scoliosis. This book will give you a clear understanding of how and why the psoas is involved with all of these issues.

THE PSOAS AND BREATHING

In addition to bridging the legs and the trunk, your psoas is intimately connected to breathing, as the diaphragm muscle, the main muscle of respiration, has ligaments that wrap around the top of the psoas and two long attachments, called cru-

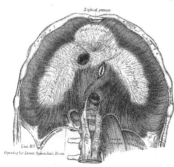

ra, that come down to insert on the first three vertebrae of the lower spine. This means that every breath resonates in some way with the psoas and the movement or lack of movement in the psoas influences each breath.

THE PSOAS AND FLEXION

The psoas is the body's main hip flexor, which is why it is the main muscle of walking, but it plays a deeper—and maybe more important role—within the nervous system. Flexors are muscles that bring one body part closer to another. The act of flexing has a relationship to the body's nervous system through our fear response. Our sympathetic nervous system, which is responsible for our flight- or-fight response, manifests through flexion; like all animals in the wild, when startled or afraid, we automatically react. The psoas is involved in any of these reactions.

Life is traumatic, and this is not necessarily a bad thing. From the big trauma of being born and taking our first breath to the lesser traumas of day-to-day life, we are here to be traumatized, and to varying degrees, we develop an inner support system to heal. Like the pulsing of the heart and the ebb and flow of the tides, the body's trauma/healing interplay is as natural as breathing.

What concerns me is when the nervous system doesn't successfully integrate a traumatic event, very often manifesting this through pain and injury to the psoas. When this happens, the trauma can become trapped in the body. This imbalance can register in many ways—emotional, postural, energetic—but it will always involve the psoas, and from my perspective, the road to relief from trauma must go through the psoas.

HOW DOES IT WORK?

The body is divisible into many systems, only some of which I will touch on here. My main concern is movement, and all movement in the body involves the skeletal system, the muscular system and the nervous system. Your bones hold you up, and your muscles move you; your nerves tell your muscles to move your bones. What we want to do is align the bones to free the nerve pathways so that they can tell the muscles to move the bones in the most efficient way. As we will see, the psoas major is intimately involved in all three of these systems.

Balance begins in the core of the body. Over the past few years, "the core" has become an abused phrase, but it deserves its due. A great deal of my interest in body mechanics stems from the complexity of our evolution from quadrupedal to bipedal beings. This shift has not been smooth.

A four-legged animal doesn't require the same balancing act from its skeleton that we do and as a result doesn't require the same core stability. It is much easier to balance a four-legged table than a two-legged table. Our ability to stand upright puts untold stresses on our muscles, bones and joints, and it is the tone and balance of the core that can and will allow for ease in the standing body.

Finding this balance requires a specific alignment of muscles and bones. For the bones to align, our muscles must have a certain amount of tone to keep everything in place.

WHY DOES IT GO WRONG?

Our posture is determined and affected by many things. In the first place, we learn by imitation, so we truly are who we come from. As we will see, the way in which we make our way to walking has a great deal of influence on our later movement pattern. Accidents, injuries and the way we heal from them often have a lasting effect on the body, as do so many other factors.

Most important is the idea that the body is a specifically designed machine in which every piece plays a part. It has been my experience that people simply don't know how they operate. Most clients that come to me are experts in something and could probably talk at length about their field. But very few can tell me exactly where or how their head is supposed to sit on top of their body. Most of us do not know that our overall health has a great deal to do with how our head sits atop our spine. The way our head sits influences our posture. And proper posture is interchangeable with proper movement and health.

Understanding the body's mechanics is a key component of our ability to institute change. If you knew that your psoas was meant to align in a specific way, and you were able to tell that the alignment felt right and seemed to take stress off your legs or back, you might be willing to do it. That is why a general understanding of anatomy is a key part of my approach to helping people make the necessary changes in the body.

Different reasons factor into an individual need for either stretching or releasing muscles. Hopefully, over the course of reading this book you will understand the need for both. The exercise section is geared toward releasing the psoas, but there are a few delicious stretches thrown in for when the psoas is ready to get long and strong.

And finally, your psoas is the tenderloin or filet mignon. In a quadruped, the psoas isn't really called on to work that much, as it doesn't actually touch the pelvis. Its function as a support structure really comes into play when tension is brought to it as we stand up and the psoas is pulled taut over the rim of the pelvis.

The distinction between quadrupedal and bipedal animals is very interesting. The evolution from being four-legged creatures to two-legged ones has not been particularly successful. And it is something that we must deal with in an effort to prevent our bodies from breaking down as we move through our 80 to 100 years.

Homo sapien is the name of our genus. This translates as "the one who knows he knows." I love that translation because I think it is our knowing that gives us so much trouble. An animal in the wild does not suffer trauma in the same way that we do.

It is our conscious thinking that allows the trauma to live in the body the way it does.

Homo sapien is only 200,000 years old. We are very young and just starting to figure these things out. I'd like to think that if we're around for another 100,000 years, we might just get this psoas and standing thing right.

Chapter II

THE PSOAS IN INFANCY

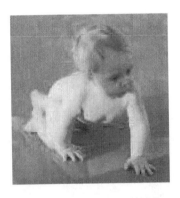

Allow me a word or two about babies. It is so easy to see the little blobs that lie before us as just that. Cute little blobs to be cooed at and passed around for others to see. But they are so much more than that. The newborn brain is developing at a rapid pace, and physical development in the first year profoundly affects us for the rest of our life.

There are many specific physical markers all babies are meant to hit along the road to standing and walking.

The journey that we all take to become a standing individual imprints many patterns that might never go away. These patterns take hold through repetition, and if we don't think at some point about changing them, there is no reason why they won't be ours forever. If you buy into that idea, we should take some time and look at the process of early development and the awakening of the psoas, which is not called upon to work until you begin to sit up and stand. In a baby's first six months, the psoas lies dormant because the legs do not bear weight, and it is actually important that they don't at this time.

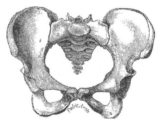

NINE IN, NINE OUT

There is a school of thought that says we are born premature—about nine months too soon—but we have to come out because the head and brain are growing too big for the human pelvis. In the process of being born, there is a big head that has to get through a little pelvis. While your bones are pretty soft as a baby, the bones of the cranium are separate, and they overlap with each other when you're born. If you touch the head of a week-old baby, you can usually feel the ridges of the cranium before they separate into a flat head.

The adult pelvis is made up of four bones: the two hip bones, the sacrum, and the coccyx, or tail bone. In utero, the pelvis contains anywhere from 12 to 14 bones. The hip bones in utero, and for about anywhere from nine months to a year after birth, are each made up of three separate bones (the ilium, the ischium and the pubis).

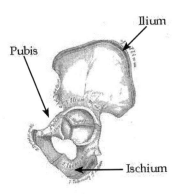

Over the course of the first year, these three bones, which meet up directly in the center of the cup (acetabulum) that the leg bone sits in, fuse.

But if these three bones haven't fused into one bone yet and you put weight on the foot and then take that weight up into that hip bone, you're not doing it a service. The hip is not designed to bear weight until those bones fuse into one solid structure. I bring this up to elucidate a very important aspect of baby handling. Babies should never be stood up on their legs until they are ready to stand by themselves.

The neighborhood where we have our yoga studio is baby central. Walk into a restaurant and it is a given that you will see parents with children, very often young babies, being stood up on their feet and held aloft by their hands. I'm not one to proselytize in restaurants, but the friends to whom I have discreetly mentioned this always say how much it seems that their babies love this feeling. It is hard to argue with the look of glee that is on their faces. It must be an amazing feeling to be standing on your parents' thighs and be at Mommy and Daddy's eye level.

Imagine, though, if you didn't stand your child up until he or she could stand on their own. After about a year (give or take) of sitting, crawling and exploring, a child will pull himself up to stand for the first time on a solid hip and confident footing.

This is all a key part of natural psoas development. Allowing the body to develop naturally is a key ingredient of coordination and grace in adulthood. Newborns should really spend as much time on their belly as possible when not being held, and babies should be allowed to find their movement markers on their own. The act of sitting up is one of life's first and most important achievements. How great would it be if children could find their way there on their own?

There is an emotional component to this process. Let's say a baby who has never been sat up finally— at around six months—sits on its own. It knows how it got there and in turn knows how to move back to square one. The inverse is that the sat-up baby has little control over its fate.

Now, these are pet peeves of mine, but they are connected to the intrinsic development of the psoas. As mentioned earlier, the psoas lies dormant in infancy and awakens in the baby's first movement from hands and knees to sitting. For many babies, sitting up and beginning to crawl often coincide.

And crawling is the next key phase in psoas development. With crawling comes the lengthening and toning that prepare the muscles to help the bones bear weight as the young skeleton makes its first forays into the world of standing. There is a similar emotional connection for babies on their bellies as opposed to babies on their backs. A baby on its belly is a grounded object—it might not be able to crawl yet, but it can touch finger and toes to the floor and have a grounded sense of a protected umbilicus. Babies on their backs are kind of lost in space, unable to do anything but flail their hands and feet to no avail.

Babies should be left on the belly as much as possible. If you sit a baby up, it doesn't really know how it got there, and it doesn't really know how to get back onto either its back or belly. But if the baby sits up on its own at the very first moment that it can, it understands how it got there, and more importantly, it knows how to get back to where it was, so it's in a very safe and grounded place.

These movements, from the floor to sitting to crawling to standing, reflect the awakening of the psoas. Crawling before standing is particularly key, as that really develops tone and length of the psoas.

Ideally, the progression is belly to sitting up to crawling to creeping, which is walking around by holding onto furniture, and then to standing. These things can't take too long. In fact, the longer it takes, the better. The more time spent at each given stage, the more the psoas will be toned and the more prepared the bones will be to bear weight for baby's first steps.

Sitting up, standing, creeping, and finally walking create a true awakening of the psoas as a support structure, and, in many ways, it will never relax again.

Chapter III

THE PSOAS IS A PULLEY

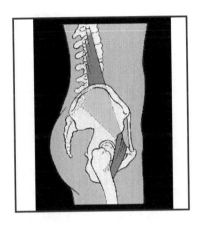

Everything changed for the psoas when we began to walk on two feet. The psoas is the filet mignon, or tenderloin, because in a quadruped it doesn't touch the pelvis during its journey from thigh to spine. When we stood up to walk on two feet, everything shifted. The big butt muscle, gluteus maximus, along with the hamstrings pulled down on the back of the pelvis to draw the spine upright. When the spine sits on top of the pelvis the psoas crosses the front rim of the pubis at the front.

As the trunk is pulled up on top of a level pelvis, the psoas tones because it attaches on the back of the inner thigh bone. The tension created in the psoas as the spine becomes vertical draws the vertebrae of the lower spine forward, effectively creating the oh-so-important lumbar curve. This small curve in the lower back, born in the ascent to bipedalism, is the weight-bearing element that allows us to stand upright and balance the rib cage and head on top of the pelvis and legs. The lumbar curve is what allows us to stand for prolonged periods of time and is one of the essential differences between humans and our nearest primate ancestors.

Once we get to standing, there are numerous opposing forces working to hold us up. We have only three muscles that connect the leg to the spine: the psoas, the piriformis and the gluteus maximus. They all attach on the thigh bone. The psoas attaches on the back of the inside of the thigh, and then it travels forward and up across the pubis. The piriformis attaches on back of the outside of the thigh and then moves slightly up to attach on the inside of the sacrum. These two muscles basically strap the spine to the leg at the front and back of the body. The piriformis muscle is often involved with pain related to the sciatic nerve (the subject of my next e-book).

Energetically, the body splits at the pelvis, with the legs rooting down to the earth and the spine lengthening to the sky. As mentioned, the gluteus maximus and hamstrings pulled down so that the spine could stand up. The psoas, which lived horizontally when we walked on all fours, is now vertical—and crucial to the spine's ability to find extension.

Also, the psoas and another group of muscles, the erector spinea muscles, interact to help the spine lengthen up. One of the things I love about anatomy is you can learn so much from looking at the names of things. The erector spinea muscles are, like the name promises, the erectors of the spine. They connect behind the psoas and run all the way up to the cranium, lengthening the spine and creating critical support for the head. These muscles work in a chain, and they all need to be able to work together for effective use.

When the psoas engages to pull the lumbar vertebrae forward, the erector spinea respond by lengthening up the back. When one or both of the psoas become tight, pulling the lower back forward into too much of a curve, the erector muscles shorten and lose tone. When these lower erectors lose tone, the upper erectors lose tone as well. This can create compression in the bones of the lower spine and can also lead to kyphosis, a common rounding of the upper back (sometimes referred to as a dowager's hump). Ideally, when the inner thigh pulls back and the tension is brought across the front rim of the pelvis, the downward pull of the front of the spine will allow an upward pull of the erectors, a counterbalancing action that provides support up through the head and the neck.

In general, a key to a healthy body is finding the balance between flexion and extension. The back muscles of the body are extensors (gluteus maximus, erector spinea); they provide extension that helps us to stand and lengthen up. The front muscles of the body (including the psoas) are flexors; they provide contraction that enables us to walk, run and survive (flexors connect to our fight-or-flight response in the nervous system). As we will soon see, most of us have this balance backward, living with posture that has basically reversed the body's natural order.

Figuring out how to successfully employ all of these muscles will allow for the body to begin to work as it was designed. The body is a machine, a series of arches, hinges and pulleys, and the psoas fits into the mechanical model as a pulley. When the psoas contracts, pulling across the front rim of the pelvis, the hip bone can act as the pulley which supports movement and change of direction. When the tight, weak or misaligned psoas fails to create this tension, lower-back pain may arise as the lumbar vertebrae are pulled forward and become compressed in the back.

The psoas is the rope, and the hip bone is the pulley. But the psoas has to be properly aligned for the pulley system to work, and in that respect the psoas must live in the back plane of the body.

The power of the psoas is based on its placement. Unfortunately, it can't place itself properly on its own. In fact, certain muscles (which we will

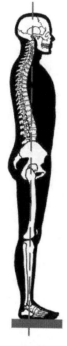

look at in the next chapter) must be toned for the psoas to be perfectly positioned.

Ideally, we can stand with good posture, as seen in the diagram on the left. This means the legs are aligned under the hips, and the head and shoulders are stacked above the hips. Then your psoas can act as a pulley.

In doing so, the psoas provides for the reciprocal upward lift of the erector spinea muscles that lengthen the spine up the back.

However, for many of us, the thighs sink forward, pulling the pelvis down at the back. Does the diagram on the right look familiar? You can see that the lower back shortens as the upper back falls backward to compensate. Welcome to 98 percent of the people who come to me for help. In this position, the psoas is drawn slightly forward and open at its base, thus losing any tension that a pulley system might provide.

Remember that the back of the body contains the extensors and the front body has the flexors. Well, when we look at the two pictures above, you can see that the guy on the left embodies this balance, while the guy on the right has actually turned his flexors into extensors and his extensors into flexors.

Stand up and take note of your posture to get a feeling for the way you normally stand. Odds are the muscles of your thighs and butt are working way more than they need to. 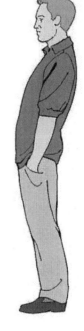 Stand with your feet parallel and try to shift your thighs backwards releasing your butt and untucking the pelvis slightly. Try and imagine how this action moves the psoas into the back plane of the body. Turn the feet out and tuck the pelvis under again and see where the insertion of the psoas goes.

It moves to the front plane of the body. When this happens, there is no longer any tension created by the pull of psoas over the rim of the pelvis, and the support offered by the pulley action disappears.

Play with this and see if you can feel the difference in the support of the spine with the butt tucked under and the feet splayed out against the reverse of sticking the butt out and turning the feet in. Feel free to exaggerate in both directions to get a feeling for what you are doing. It is great to do this in front of a mirror and watch for the effect on the body. With the butt tucked under and the thighs sinking forward, the lower back collapses, as does the neck, forcing the head slightly forward. Stick your butt out and see the difference as the lower back and neck both lengthen in a good way, bringing support to the spine.

Every time you find the proper placement of the pelvis, you are feeling the power of the psoas. And that feeling is the pulley action as the inner thigh pulls down and the psoas draws the lumbar spine forward allowing the spinal muscle to lengthen the spine to vertical.

From my perspective, this most common misalignment—thighs leaning forward, pulling the psoas into the front plane of the body— is responsible for a great deal of our shoulder, head and neck soreness. Fortunately, developing the action of the psoas as a pulley is a relatively easy way to help ourselves find proper standing alignment.

Chapter IV

MUSCLES THAT SUPPORT THE PSOAS

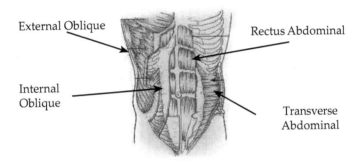

External Oblique

Rectus Abdominal

Internal Oblique

Transverse Abdominal

THE HOLY TRINITY

Our bones hold us up, and our muscles move us. I am always trying to simplify and reduce things to easily understood sound bites. But it is often more complicated. In this section, we are going to look at three muscle groups, the holy trinity, that work to support the ideal positioning of the psoas. For the psoas to be the wonder muscle that it is designed to be, it must be properly situated at its top and bottom, and it can't find that placement by itself.

These groups are the adductors, muscles of the inner thigh; the levator ani, muscles of the pelvic floor; and the eight abdominal muscles.

THE INNER THIGHS

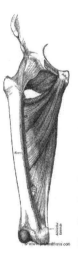

The adductors, the inner-thigh muscles, move the leg in toward the midline, and they help stabilize the pelvis. There are five of them. The shortest of them is the pectinius, which attaches high up on the inner thigh and into the pelvis. The gracilis attaches to the pelvis and all the way down to the shin. And the three middle ones are adductor magnus, longus and brevis.

All of these muscles attach around the pubic bone. But the adductor magnus, the biggest of them, has one head that attaches to one of your sit bones, the ischeal tuboroscity. Interestingly, that makes this muscle responsible for not just moving your leg to the midline but also assisting with internal rotation.

And that ability to rotate the leg in is an absolute key to stabilizing and setting the psoas.

Proper tone of the adductors allows for the psoas to live in the back plane of the body, which, as we've seen already, is vital to good posture.

MUSCLE BALANCE

Let's take a moment to look at the concept of muscle balance. Every group of muscles has an

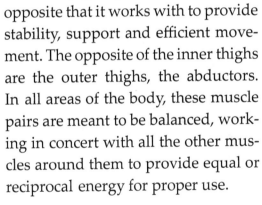

opposite that it works with to provide stability, support and efficient movement. The opposite of the inner thighs are the outer thighs, the abductors. In all areas of the body, these muscle pairs are meant to be balanced, working in concert with all the other muscles around them to provide equal or reciprocal energy for proper use.

There are classic imbalances resulting from poor posture due to the unsuccessful employment of the psoas. In the neck, one of the most common misalignments—the ears being forward of the shoulders—creates a strong imbalance between muscles on the front and back of the neck. Most people tend to be closed in the front of their upper chest, so those muscles are short and tight and the back muscles are long and weak.

It starts at the base of the body—if the shin-bones and calves settle backward, the thighs are forced forward, drawing the pelvis down and causing the lower back to shorten (no pulley). As a result, the upper back falls backward and the upper chest rounds in, taking the head and neck with it.

We are supposed to be evenly balanced, with the upper chest as equally wide and broad as the upper back. Our inner and outer thighs have their own reasons why they are rarely a happy couple. One of them returns us to early childhood. Just as sitting up and crawling awaken the psoas, these movements also are a significant vehicle for inner-thigh development.

Crawling employs a dynamic stretching of the psoas and optimal use of the young adductor muscles. If employed over a length of time, when a baby pulls him- or herself up to stand, there will be beautiful balance and tone between the inner and outer thigh. To this end, it is not in a baby's interest to walk early. In fact, barring neurological problems, the longer a baby crawls the better, allowing time for the growth of core coordination. But crawling is only one issue.

POSTURAL IMBALANCE

Very few of us are aligned to allow for balance between the inner and outer thighs. If you tend to stand and walk with your feet turned out, which I'd say is a large part of the population, your inner thigh would by necessity be weaker than the outer thigh—due to the position of the foot and pelvis, the inner leg turns out and is no longer in a position to work effectively.

Many of us stand this way because our parents stood this way, and so much of our learning is by imitation. Unfortunately, generation after generation of bad posture will haunt us until we get it right.

Think about your parents and siblings and try to figure out whose posture and body type you inherited, if one more than the other. Figure out who you move and walk like and then try to de-cipher why that might be the case. It might not be a parent.

It could be an older sibling that you bonded with or an aunt whom you loved dearly. That which we become is a tapestry of so many threads.

So what does this imbalance bring us? Outer-thigh dominance tends to pull us toward external rotation, which really complicates things. Your deep gluteal muscles are designed to function as both internal and external rotators. The problem is that these designs are based on the ideal. Should you stand up straight and have both feet pointing forward and not too far apart, the gluteals would be positioned in such a way that they could serve both functions. Half of their span would be to-ward the front plane of the body, and half would be toward the back.

Try standing with the feet together, the eyes closed, and the big buttock muscle, gluteus maxi-mus, relaxed, and see if you can sense what is go-ing on deep inside. The gluteals are dynamically going back and forth in search of a stable place between inner and outer rotation. Now turn the feet out and move them apart. It is likely that the pelvis shuts down energetically, its joints become somewhat locked, and the inner rotation of the thighs, which is always key to the psoas, is gone.

Building proper tone in the inner thighs is imperative if we want to get our legs under our pelvis for proper posture. The psoas can't live in the back plane of the body without the help of balanced leg muscles.

THE PELVIC FLOOR

The muscles of the pelvic floor are called the levator ani. Three muscles form a sling at the bottom of the pelvis that connects the tailbone to the pubis. This mass of muscle, about the thickness of your palm, is responsible for holding the pelvic organs in place and for control of rectal and urogenital function. Not only are these muscles bearing a lot of weight from above; they are also pierced by orifices that weaken the pelvic floor merely by their presence. Continence is high on my list of priorities, and the pelvic floor and continence are dancing partners that we must train and respect. Because these muscles are involved with your eliminative functioning, they have more resting tone than any other muscle in the body and are almost always active—or you'd be peeing all night long.

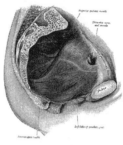

The pelvis and the muscles surrounding it serve a role unique to bipedal mammals. Just like the psoas, which is relatively dormant in quadrupeds (hence the tenderness of its loin) but wakes up when standing upright brings it into positive tension across the rim of the pelvis, the pelvic floor has a greatly different role in the biped. If you think of a dog, a cat or a horse, their pelvis is the back wall of the body rather than the floor. This leaves the organs in a dog to rest on the belly. In standing bipeds, the organs sit right on top of this muscle group, which frankly has enough to do without its newfound responsibility. Kegels exercises were created to help women with post-pregnancy incontinence issues. I think these exercises are the most important exercises any of us can do (we will learn to build the inner thighs and do Kegels in the third e-book in this series).

When you have strength in the pelvic floor muscles, what you're getting is a stable pelvis, and the stability of the pelvis allows for the psoas to move across the rim of the pelvis and have a proper, strong and toned gliding action on its journey to being a pulley.

When you have strength in the pelvic floor, what you're getting is a stable pelvis, and the stability of the pelvis allows for the psoas to move across the rim of the pelvis and have a proper, strong, toned gliding action on its journey to being a pulley.

THE ABS

Muscles of the Trunk

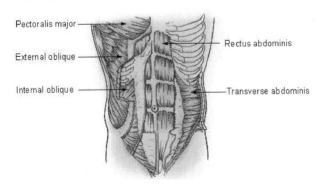

The last group of muscles we'll look at is the abdominals, equally important for many different reasons. You have eight abdominal muscles— four pairs. All four sets of these muscles move in different directions.

As we look at a cross section of the trunk (below), notice the way the abdominal muscles are all connected, both through the tendons and the fascia.

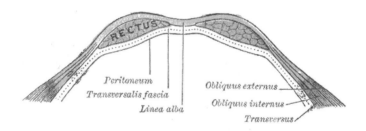

The deepest of them is the transverse abdominus. It wraps from the back to the front, meeting at the linea alba. We often refer to the transverse as one muscle, but it is two muscles that meet in the middle. This deep muscle when properly toned, provides a great deal of support to the lumbar spine.

The next layer of abdominal muscles consists of the internal and external obliques, which are angled in opposite directions. These muscles help in twisting, rotating, bending and flexing the trunk and are also active when we exhale.

THE SIX-PACK

The third set of abs is the rectus abdominus, the "six-pack." This pair of muscles runs vertically, connecting at the pubis at its base and the sternum and three ribs at its top. An anatomical aside about the six-pack: the body has interesting and different ways of compensating for dilemmas of length and space. The length between the pelvis and the rib cage is really too big for one long muscle to provide support. As a result we have tendinous insertions that fall between what are actually ten small muscles. So we really build ten-packs, but we only see six of them. This pack is formed when we make these individual muscles big enough so that they essentially pop out from the tendons that surround them. Muscle is designed to stretch; tendons are not.

HARD MUSCLE IS BAD

I have a clear image in my head of the guy on

TV selling his six-minute abs program. He looks out at the camera with his six-pack jutting proud, but his shoulders are hunched over toward his pelvis as though he couldn't stand up straight if he wanted to. I always wonder if he is bent over to make his muscles pop or if that is his natural and proud posture.

I guess this might look good to some, but I'd like to take a moment to explain the nature of what happens to your muscles as you build them. Blood flows into muscles, passing through the endless number of fibers that make up an individual muscle.

The way we build muscle is by creating micro tears in the muscle fibers; as they heal or repair, the body overcompensates in a way, replacing the damaged tissue and adding more, for protection against further damage. As we continue to build a muscle, the fibers need to have somewhere to go, and they begin laying down on top of one another. As more mass develops, the layering becomes denser and harder. At a certain density, blood flow will begin to become inhibited.

Just as the tight psoas results in back and other problems, a tight rectus can bring its own set of problems. Depending on the individual, breathing, digestion, circulation, and even the flow of nervous energy can be impaired.

The cultural arena of our body is a fascinating one. We have so many compensatory patterns due to the way we feel and look. We tuck our pelvis because we think our butt is too big, we hunch our shoulders to hide our breasts or because we don't like being tall. There are many more to add to this list, but I am really fascinated by the desire for six- pack abs. Our society lives in worship of the sit-up or crunch, thinking it is an express train to beauty.

Whether you think they are beautiful or not doesn't matter compared to knowing what they do and how they are connected to all of the other abdominal muscles. When we look at the cross section again it should become clear that because these muscles are connected to one another, they need to have equal tone. Imagine if one set were way stronger than the other, as tends to be the case with the rectus abdominus: as one muscle gets stronger, the other groups become weaker. We have to step back to find a new approach to balanced muscle building.

The fact that every muscle is designed to carry out a specific function has little bearing on what that muscle actually does. The brain might have a wish list in terms of a nervous response to a given stimulus, but a dominant muscle will take over ten out of ten times. With regard to the abs, it is the rectus abdominus that tends to engage at the expense of all the other abdominals.

These abs aid in breathing and help all movements of the trunk and pelvis, and for the purpose of the psoas they go a long way toward stabilizing the vertebrae and reducing stress on the spine.

Hopefully you are beginning to see that if these muscles are connected, they need to have equal tone. If they don't, and one of the four groups is stronger than the other, the other three groups are going to get weaker. The other, more pleasant scenario is that it is almost guaranteed that your psoas can find its proper place if these three muscle groups, the holy trinity of the inner thighs, pelvic floor and the abdominals, are toned and living in their proper places.

Chapter V

THE EFFECTS OF A TIGHT PSOAS

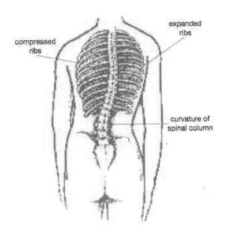

A happy psoas major is a long muscle that lives deep in the bowl of the pelvis, creating a shelf of sorts for the abdominal contents on both sides of the body.

Let's begin our journey into dysfunction by tightening the psoas on the right side. Everyone is tighter on one side of the body—stronger and tighter on one side and looser and weaker on the other; they both have their advantages and disadvantages.

Let's see what happens when the right psoas tightens. The right leg is pulled up into the right hip, restricting movement. The psoas has a bit of external rotation when it is flexed, and this shows up in the tight hip by turning out the right foot. Another possibility is that the tight psoas both pulls the right hip up and draws the bottom rib down.

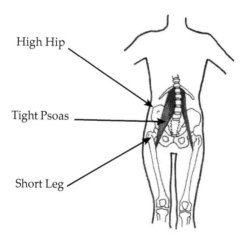

High Hip

Tight Psoas

Short Leg

Have you ever noticed that one of your legs is shorter than the other? Almost everybody is going to fall into this category. But maybe one in a million people actually has shorter bones on one leg shorter than the other. Most often it is the tightness of the psoas muscle that creates this discrepancy in leg length.

It is easy to go through life and never even realize that one of your legs is shorter than the other, and some people find out about it in odd ways, like going to a tailor and when their pants come back hemmed they see that one leg is shorter than the other.

How well do you know your posture? Does one of your legs turn out more than the other? If it does, that too is likely the pull of a tight psoas.

Beyond leg-length discrepancy there is an endless array of dysfunctional possibilities for the psoas. Imagine if both psoas are tight. What will happen in this case is the femurs get jammed up into the hip socket, and the psoas pulls the lumbar vertebrae too far forward, creating an excessive curve. And that excessive lumbar curve finds compensation in what's called a kyphosis, where the upper back pulls in opposition to the lower back.

I see this pattern in 75 percent of my clients to one degree or another.

A tight psoas on one side means that the leg on that side will be pulled tight into the hip socket.

This is one of the hallmarks of what we in yoga call tight hips. The psoas isn't the only contributor to tight hips, but it is almost always involved. Any time there is this kind of environment in the hips, movement is going to be restricted, and the leg and pelvis will tend to move as a unit rather than moving independently as designed. Functional movement in our body is dependent on freely moving joints. And the movement in our joints is reciprocal with other joints in the body. There are specific correlations between the hips and the ankles and the knees and the lower back. If the movement at the hip is restricted, as it will be with a tight psoas, that movement is going to have to come from some other joints, and this is one of the reasons why we have such a high incidence of knee and lumbar injuries. Movement that should occur in the pelvis and hips comes either from above or below and negatively affects those joints.

Many people believe that scoliosis is due to

shortness or tightness in the psoas. Let's take a look at how that might work. You have the psoas on two sides, but imagine if only one is tight. If I pull down on this psoas, it's very easy to see how the pelvis might twist and torque forward. As a result of the pelvis twisting and torquing, the rest of the spine is going to have to twist along with it—there's really no way to avoid that.

Besides the spine moving, another result will be that muscles begin to move in opposition; even ribs can get involved. In a really bad case of scoliosis you might see that the upper ribs are so affected that you get what appears to be a hunch-back as the ribs are pulled back.

Compensation is possibly the most important part of understanding and unraveling what it is we're trying to do in the body. If my car breaks down, that's it—it doesn't go anywhere. If I get a flat tire, I'm stuck with my flat until I get my flat fixed. But if my body breaks down, it is designed to compensate.

The muscle that compensates, unfortunately, has to take on a lesser role in its original function and often can't work as well because it is doing two jobs rather than one. If I hurt the inside of my foot, the muscles of the inside of my foot do not work as well, and the muscles of the outside of my foot have to help. That, by nature, is going to diminish the quality of the muscles of the outside of the foot.

That is going on everywhere, but it's not such a bad thing if we heal and then reverse the course of compensation. But we are rarely that conscious, and very often these compensatory patterns become part of the body and stay part of the body.

If you start to learn about your body and how it works, you come to understand the power of the psoas and realize how opening, stretching and releasing it can bring amazing health to the body; then there's a real incentive to find this health.

Chapter VI

THE PSOAS AND THE ORGANS

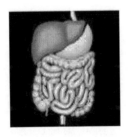

The psoas exerts a great influence on the contents of the trunk. When you have a long and toned psoas, it lives down in the bowl of the pelvis, and it creates a container for the organs with the pelvic floor below, the rectus abdominus in front and the diaphragm above providing support and protection for everything within.

The contents of the trunk, your organs, should live in or above the bowl of the pelvis. A short, tight psoas gets in the way of this possibility. The tightness of the psoas pulls the lumbar vertebrae and the psoas forward. If the abdominal muscles lack tone, the trunk's contents are pushed forward; if there is too much tone, they can get squished in between the psoas and the strong abs.

Have you ever seen a pregnant woman who is so big that she looks like she's going to have twins yet she is carrying an average-sized baby? The fetus and the abdominal contents can be pushed forward due to psoas tightness, and it might appear that she is going to have a giant baby.

Have you ever seen a skinny person who has a potbelly, but they don't have a lot of fat on their body? Again, the tightness of the psoas can push the abdominal contents forward, resulting in the appearance of a potbelly.

WALKING IS FALLING

We often come back to the psoas as the main muscle of walking. When we are functioning correctly, the entire body is toned and stimulated by proper walking pattern. When you learn how to walk properly, the body's natural healing processes can kick into gear.

Walking is a core event initiated by the nervous system in response to falling. Let's say the right leg is in front as you are moving forward through space. The brain tells the psoas of the back or left leg to initiate movement to catch you before you fall. Walking is, at its core, falling endlessly forward through life trying to find yourself in the effortless wave of gravity's flow.

Instead of that ideal, most of us tend to walk or fall backward, leading with the legs, placing the feet down ahead of you, instead of falling forward through the feet. This pattern fails to take advantage of the psoas during walking.

Walking from the psoas initiates a spinal twist with each step that is facilitated by the alternating movement of the arms and the legs. When the right leg and hip go forward the right arm releases backward. At the same time, the left leg and hip go backward and the left arm goes forward. This results in a spinal twist with every step that allows for and encourages the proper movement in the pelvis and spinal joints, twists and cleanses the internal organs, and affords better access to the breath through a more effective interplay of the psoas and diaphragm. One of the key benefits of the FitzGordon Method core walking program

is wellness through movement. Good gait is pre-
ventative medicine.

When your psoas begins to walk you through
life, it is drawn down and back through the inner
thigh. Your lumbar spine is pulled forward. When
you switch legs, the opposite happens. Add the
arms to that, because the arms and the legs move
in symmetrical opposition, and you get a powerful rotation through the lumbar spine that is stimulated and initiated by the psoas.

This aff everything in the area. Very specific, it
stimulates and massages the intestines and the
bladder and really begins to show you the connection of the psoas to digestive and eliminative
health.

The psoas lives right next door to the bladder.

Many people wake up to urinate a lot of times
over the course of a night. Very often, it is a short,
tight psoas pressing against the bladder that
creates the environment for that to happen, and
hopefully releasing can help you alleviate that.

A short and tight psoas can also restrict the
flow of blood and create circulation problems.

The abdominal aorta, which supplies blood to the pelvis abdomen and legs, splits into the left and right iliac arteries which follow the path of the psoas down towards the leg. Poor circulation in the feet and toes can be a common indicator of psoas problems.

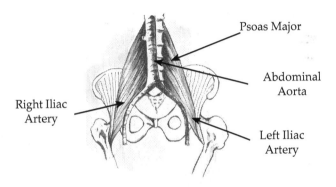

Psoas Major

Abdominal Aorta

Right Iliac Artery

Left Iliac Artery

Let's look at the psoas's connection to breath and the diaphragm, which can have a profound effect on the nervous system. Fascia, ligaments and tendons all connect the diaphragm and the psoas.

There are two tendons, called crura, which come down from the diaphragm to attach on the lumbar spine alongside the psoas attachments; the ligament of the diaphragm wraps around the top of the psoas, where it connects into the 12th thoracic vertebra These connections mean that the psoas is involved with every breath and the diaphragm is involved with every step.

The pelvic floor and the diaphragm are synergistic. What that means is that they work together. Every time you inhale, and this is in a healthy, ideal body, the pelvic floor and the diaphragm both lower fractionally. And they both rise with every exhale.

Connect this to the breath and the synergistic working of the diaphragm and the pelvic floor, and you start to get a really amazing bit of movement in the body. With every inhale the psoas draws back into the bowl of the pelvis as the rectus abdominus draws forward, and the diaphragm and pelvic floor lower. With every exhale everything retracts, the diaphragm and the pelvic floor move up, and the psoas and the rectus draw back in.

This gives us a window into the work of the psoas as a hydraulic pump in concert with the synchronized pumping of the diaphragm and the pelvic fl. This stimulates and massages all the organs and all the bones and moves fluids through the entire trunk.

Chapter VII

THE PSOAS AND THE NERVOUS SYSTEM

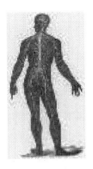

The nervous system is the body's information gatherer, storage center, and control system. It collects info, analyzes it and initiates the proper response. The central nervous system, which is the big kahuna, includes the brain and spinal cord.

The peripheral nervous system connects the central nervous system to the body via nerves that come out of the central nervous system.

There are a number of divisions within the nervous system. Your peripheral nervous system has a motor division, and within that motor division, there are two other divisions, the somatic and the autonomic systems. Within the autonomic systems come two subsystems that we will focus on.

These are the sympathetic nervous system and the parasympathetic nervous system. The sympathetic is the system of excitation, and the parasympathetic is the system of relaxation. Both systems innervate the same organs and act in opposition to maintain homeostasis, the Greek word for staying stable or staying the same. For example, when you are scared, the sympathetic system causes your heart to beat faster; when the fear has passed, the parasympathetic system reverses this effect. Homeostasis, the search for balance between excitation and relaxation, is at the heart of our well- being.

We move now from the purely mechanical workings of the psoas and dive into its deeper role in the body.

We know that nerves tell muscles to move bones. But there is also an emotional side as well; the nervous system is constantly working to maintain harmony in the realm of fear, worry and safety. The fear response plays a large role in our movement and postural capabilities. The main action of this response is flexion, so we return always to the psoas, the body's main hip flexor. Any time we are involved with the sympathetic nervous system, the psoas will be involved, which is fine as long as the journey into fear is balanced by an alternate response from the parasympathetic system.

Life is fear, and our relationship to fear is a large part of what determines the nature of our health, our posture, our muscle tone, even our emotional tone—maybe especially our emotional tone. And fear is flexion. We flex for security; we flex because we need to in reaction to the fears that come up in life. It doesn't matter what these actions of safety or protection are—running, fighting, hiding—they're all flexion.

And we always come back to the psoas. All of these acts of flexion are great if they're balanced by a happy interaction with the parasympathetic nervous system. They're designed to work together.

Let me give you an example of the interaction of these two systems. Let's say it's the middle of August and you walk outside onto the street and it's 100 degrees. The first thing that happens is your internal body temperature begins to rise. As that happens, your nervous system takes note, and the sympathetic nervous system kicks into action to produce sweat to cool down the body and reduce internal temperature.

As soon as the body temperature is lowered, the parasympathetic nervous system comes into play to reduce the sweat. This happy interplay is constantly going on in your body. Let's say you cooled down enough to stop sweating but then get on an air-conditioned bus. The same mini drama plays out in the nervous system, seeking balance of the internal environment.

What concerns us is when something creates an imbalance between these two systems. This imbalance can register emotionally, posturally, or energetically, but it will always involve the psoas, and from my perspective, the road to relief from trauma must go through the psoas.

Now I'll share a story of what it is like to get

stuck in the sympathetic nervous system. Let's say you have a boss whom you hate, but you have to see him every day at work. You get in the car in the morning at 8:00 and settle in for the hour's drive to work. Life is good. You listen to the radio, maybe talk on the phone. You're feeling good.

As soon as you get to work, you pull into the parking lot and shut the ignition off, and all of a sudden you feel the engagement of the sympathetic nervous system. Maybe it's a little white light across your lower back; maybe it's a tingling up and down your spine; maybe your mouth goes dry. Whatever it is, you're no longer happy. You have just gone from ease to dis-ease.

But that's okay, because you and your boss work in different areas in the office. You pass by his office, you say hello, he grunts hello and you relax a little—the parasympathetic steps in, says, Oh, okay, we can bring balance back, let's chill out.

You have to do it again at lunch, and you have to do it again when you leave work, but that's all right, that's the natural process, the natural balance. But let's change the scenario a little bit and say that your boss does not have a separate office and you work at a desk next to him. What happens then?

At 9:00 a.m., the car turns off, and the sympathetic nervous system turns on and does not release until you leave. You walk on eggshells, and everything that happens during the day creates a startle response. You're always waiting for that reaction. You're always waiting in fear, and as a result the sympathetic nervous system stays engaged and will never release.

This story can be applied to many different scenarios, most profoundly to war zones, car accidents, destructive home environments, muggings, etc. Any trauma can create this imbalance in the nervous system. The specific event or trauma doesn't matter. It is the body's ability to process the trauma that determines what comes next. Essentially it is the body's ability to discharge the trauma that allows for a healthy fear response and in turn a better chance to achieve homeostasis, which is where the psoas release comes in. The body, when traumatized, will process the trauma, but it can't always process it immediately and it can't always process it well.

To release the psoas is to allow for a letting-go of long-held trauma, whatever that trauma might be.

If the stuff of our lives is still living in the body, we want to try to come up with a way of letting it go. And for me, releasing the psoas is the key first step on a long journey to a balanced body. It has been my experience that you can't stretch a muscle that is full of tension, whether that tension is postural or emotional. You must first learn to step back and release these muscles before you can dive into a beautiful journey of building length and tone in free and easy muscles.

Chapter VIII

RELEASES

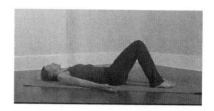

WHAT IS A RELEASE?

The exercises in this manual are as much about exploring your psoas and your pelvis—specifically your pelvis's relation to the legs as they meet the hip sockets and the sacrum where it meets the lumbar spine—as they are about healing. With the FitzGordon Method, healing cannot begin without awareness. Settle into these explorations to come to a better understanding of how your body works.

Physical, emotional and postural health are predicated on a body having supple joints. We are essentially drying up from the moment we are born, and a great deal of our struggle in aging is about staying lubricated. Tight, constricted joints inhibit lubrication. Again, if you are reading this you likely have some tight joints. Every one of these releases is intended to bring movement and clarity to the hip joint.

Finally, before you begin, know that releases are about not doing. Want less and you will get more.

Trauma is a strange bedfellow. It has no interest in hanging around. You just have to find the subtle means of letting it leave.

The following exercises can be done in sequence if you have the time but are also effectve individually. For instance, someone who experiences hip pain while walking can stop on any street corner to do the Foot on a Block exercise that comes third in this series. Temporary relief can go a long way toward permanent relief when it comes to retraining the nervous system to believe that pain can be abated.

What you will need:

- A mat.

- A belt.

- A blanket.

- Three yoga blocks or equivalent-size books.

- A tennis ball.

- An orange or its equivalent

CONSTRUCTIVE REST POSITION (CRP)

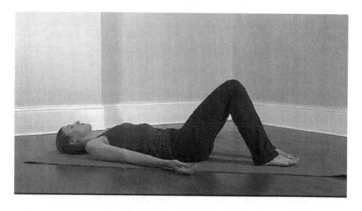

This is the main psoas release that we work on. It is a gravitational release of the psoas that allows the force of gravity to have its way with the contents of the trunk and the deep core.

- Lie on your back with your knees bent and your heels situated 12 to 16 inches away from your pelvis, in line with your sit bones.

- You can tie a belt around the middle of the thighs. This is a good thing to do, especially if you are weak in the inner thighs. You want to be able to really let go here and not have to think too much about the position of your legs.

- Then do nothing. You want to allow the body to let whatever happens to it come and go. Discomfort arises from conditioned muscular patterns. Try to allow the body to release rather than shift or move when unpleasant sensations arise.

- You are hoping to feel sensation that is something you can sit with and allow to pass.

- Try to do this for 15 minutes a day, twice a day—in the morning and at night. If you have time, longer sessions are advisable.

But we are not here to suffer. If sensations come up and you feel that you just have to move, feel free to move, then come back to where you were and try again. It's possible that you'll do this exercise and not feel anything; that is fine also.

TENNIS BALL UNDER FOOT

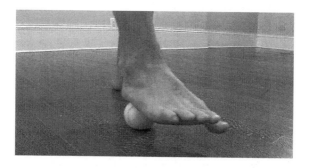

Technically, this is not a psoas release, but it is a gift to the body any way you look at it. This is great before or after constructive rest as well as anytime during the day. I recommend keeping a tennis ball in a shoe box under your desk; that will keep the ball from escaping away while you roll.

- Place a tennis ball under your right foot.

- Spend a minute or two rolling the ball under the foot. You can be gentle, or you can apply more pressure. The choice is yours.

Step off of the tennis ball and bend over your legs. You can check in with your body and see if you feel that the right leg seems a bit longer and looser. Feel free to scan the whole body in this fashion.

There is a thick pad of connective tissue on the sole of the foot called the plantar fascia. By releasing the fascia on the underside of the right foot, you effectively release the entire right side of the body.

FOOT ON A BLOCK

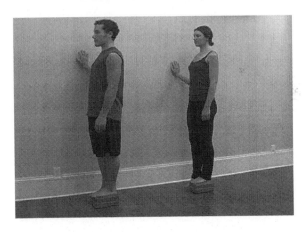

This is a gravitational release of the psoas. This exercise is not limited to your house. If you have hip or groin pain when walking, feel free to stop at every corner and dangle one foot off of the curb while holding on to a lamp post.

- Place a block eight to ten inches from a wall.

- Step the left foot up on the block, allowing the right foot to hang down between the block and the wall. Place your right arm on the wall to help you stabilize the upper body.

- Keep the hips level and rotate the inner thighs back and apart—stick out your butt a bit, and feel like you can let the leg go from the base of the rib cage, the top of the psoas. Once you are comfortable with the leg hanging out of the hip, you can move the leg half an inch forward and back as slowly and steadily as possible. Half an inch is a very short distance.

Let the leg dangle this way for 30 seconds or until the standing hip has done enough.

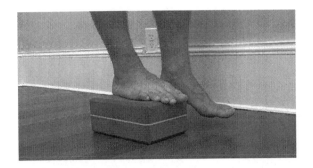

- Switch sides and tune in to which side is tighter. Do the second side for the same length of time that you did on the first side.

- Repeat for a second time on the tighter side.

DIFFERENTIATING LEG FROM TRUNK

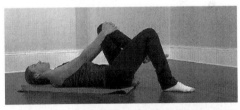

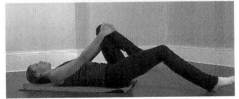

- Bend the left knee and interlace your fingers at the top of the shin. Hold the leg out at arm's length. Extend the other leg. Pay attention to the hip socket—only move your leg, not the pelvis.

- Bring tone to the pelvic floor and the low belly and do your best to stabilize the trunk.

- Extend the right leg out slowly. It doesn't have to extend completely.

- Slowly lift the right knee up, drawing the heel toward the hip and keeping the left heel on the floor with the foot flexed.

- Maintaining a stable trunk, extend the right leg out again.

- Repeat ten times on each side if possible. Feel free to start with as few as three times.

SUB OCCIPITALS

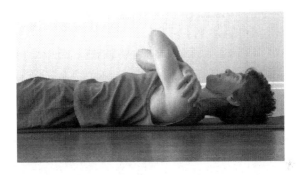

The sub occipital muscles connect the base of the skull to the top of the spine and are the only muscles in the body with an energetic connection to the eyes. They tend to be chronically short.

- Lie flat on your back and bring a small natural arch to your lower back. The legs should be straight; you can put a blanket under the knees if there is any strain on the lower back.

- Raise your arms to the sky, pulling your shoulder blades away from the floor. Try to let the upper spine settle onto the ground. Grasp each shoulder with the opposite hand.

- Lengthen the back of the neck as much as you can without closing off or creating discomfort at the front of the throat.

- Hold the position for three minutes to start, and try to build up to five minutes.

RELEASING ARM

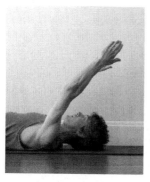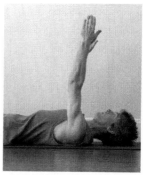

This exercise works on the ability to articulate the arms separately from the trunk.

- Start on your back with your knees bent and your feet flat on the floor.

- Reach straight arms up, with the fingers pointing toward the ceiling.

- Feel how much or how little of the ribcage is on the floor. Feel the curve or lack thereof in the lower back.

- The idea is to separate the arms and the rib-cage.

- Begin to take the arms over head towards the fl behind you keeping the arms straight and parallel.

- Feel for movement the rib cage and spine.

- If the spine moves, or the elbows bend or arms separate you have gone too far. Come back to the beginning and start again.

The goal is not to go all the way to the fl but to only move where the arm and trunk separate easily.

CACTUS

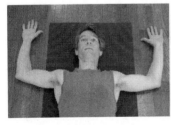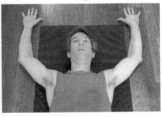

This falls somewhere between a release and a stretch and is not nearly as benign as some of these explorations. In fact, this can be very intense, though you won't be doing much.

- Lie flat on your back. If it is not comfortable to lie with the legs straight, roll up a blanket and place it under the knees. This will release the hamstrings and reduce the strain on the lower back.

- Bring your arms out to the side and bend your elbows to form a right angle with the arms.

- Lengthen the back of the neck and allow the spine to soften toward the floor. The lower back and neck should each have a gentle arch, but ideally the rest of the spine should have contact with the floor. Move very slowly.

- Once you get your spine into a good place, bring your awareness to the forearms, wrists and hands. Try to open the hands, extending the wrists and the fingers. Move very slowly.

- Once you get the arm to a good place return to the spine. Go back and forth between the two and allow the back of the body to lengthen, soften, and release.

BLOCK LUNGES

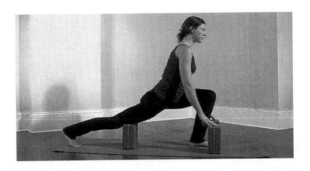

This is a release of both the quadriceps and the psoas. Sometimes the quadriceps muscles are so tight, there is no getting to the psoas until we release the quads a bit. You'll need three blocks for this.

- Positioned on your hands and knees or in Downward Facing Dog, step the right foot forward in between your hands. Two blocks will be for your hands by the front foot.

- Place the third block underneath the quadriceps muscle just above the knee, at the base of the thigh.

- Tuck the back toes and let the weight of the body fall onto the block. Do your best to keep the heel of the back foot pointing straight up toward the ceiling.

- The front leg and hip should not be under any strain. Feel free to make adjustments, turning the foot out or stepping the foot wider.

- You need to stay for 90 seconds to get the full benefits of this pose.

RELEASING HANDS AND KNEES

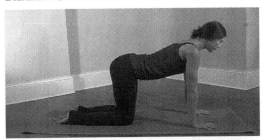

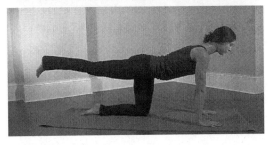

This exercise explores the ability of the leg to separate from the pelvis and the spine.

- Start on your hands and knees with the hips over the knees and the wrists underneath the shoulders.

- Bring gentle tone to the pelvic floor and the lower belly and try to extend your right leg back, bringing the leg level with the trunk.

- Keep your awareness on the lower back and the pelvis stabilizing the trunk to release the leg.

As always, these are experiential exercises where you try to get a feeling for what the body is doing.

The tighter psoas will be the side that can't move without pulling the pelvis and the spine with it.

TONING

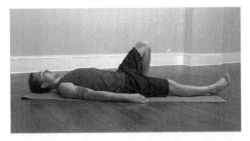

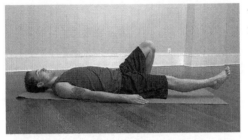

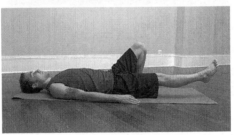

The following exercise works the psoas more than most of these explorations. Proceed slowly, and don't overdo it in the beginning.

- Begin in constructive rest. Extend the right leg straight out.

- Press the left foot down into the floor to help the right leg lift up two inches.

- Lift the right leg three or four inches higher, and then lower it back to two inches off the floor.

- Repeat five times if possible, keeping the pelvis and spine stable. The only thing working is the leg.

- Switch sides.

Once you are comfortable taking the leg up and down, begin again by pressing the opposite foot into the floor. One variation is to move the leg from side to side, and another is to move the leg on a diagonal, staying within a three- or four-inch range of motion.

Note: Three inches is a very short distance.

TIGHT-HIP RELEASE

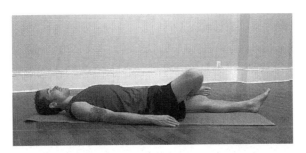

This is meant as a passive release for extreme-ly tight hips. If your knee is higher than a 45-de-gree angle from the floor when you assume this position, this exercise is for you.

- Lie on your back with the legs straight out on the floor. Stabilize the trunk and bring the right foot as high up on the left thigh as possible.

- Allow the right knee to release toward the floor, keeping the trunk stable the entire time.

- Try to let the release come from both the inner and outer thigh as gravity takes the leg toward the floor.

- Stay for five minutes on each side if possible.

ORANGE THING

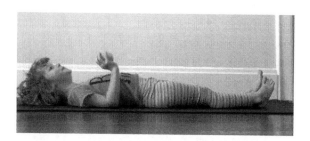

This is more for fun than anything else. Look at yourself in a mirror before and after you have done one side and see if notice a difference.

- Lay flat on your back with an orange or a ball of similar size sitting by your right hip.

- Roll the orange slowly back and forth from the heel of your palm to the fingertips.

- Pick up the orange and hold it in your open palm with the elbow on the floor and the palm facing the ceiling.

- Balance the orange on your palm for two or three minutes before stopping.

Chapter IX

STRETCHES

PSOAS STRETCH: LUNGE ON FLOOR

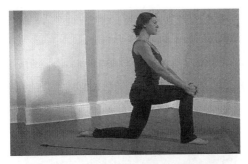

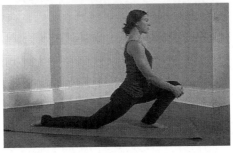

In this exercise we'll experience a dynamic stretch of the psoas.

- Start on your hands and knees and step the right foot forward in between your hands. Feel how all four corners of the trunk are pointing straight ahead. Try to maintain that alignment throughout the whole pose.*

- Interlace the fingers on the right knee. You can use the strength of the arms to help lengthen and extend the spine.

- We want the psoas to move back in space at the inner thigh and the lower back as the pelvis comes forward.

Try to wrap the inner thigh of the right leg back, feeling the outer hip come forward. Take the low spine back and up, lengthening up all the way through the back of the neck, and allow the pelvis and the front knee to come forward if possible.

- Repeat on the second side.

*If the hips are tight, you're going to feel restricted as you come forward and try to work on squaring the hips toward the front. It's okay if the hips don't square completely. Don't worry about how deep the stretch is—you don't need to go deep. You just want to explore the basic idea of keeping the hips square and stretching your psoas.

PSOAS STRETCH: STANDING

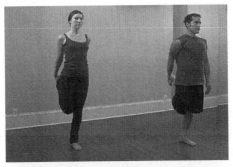

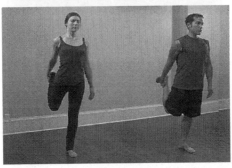

This is a classic standing stretch that also happens to be a deep stretch of the psoas—if it is done correctly. Feel free to use the wall to support yourself.

- Bend your right leg behind you and take hold of the right foot or ankle with your right hand. Bring your knees in line with one another, keeping the heel in line with your sit bone. If your outer hip is very tight it won't be easy to keep the knees in line.

- Pull the right leg behind you gently. Keep the pelvis and shoulders facing forward and upright the whole time.

- Keep the pelvic floor and the low belly strong as you try to pull the leg behind you through the balanced action of the inner and outer thigh.

If you have tight hips, it will be difficult to keep the legs aligned as you draw the right leg back. The knee will pull sideways, and it is imperative that you keep the legs in line. This is an issue with the iliotibial tract, or IT band, not the psoas, but as we know, everything is connected (no pun intended).

EXTENDED SIDE ANGLE

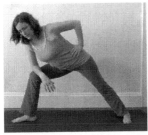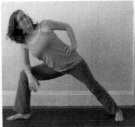

- Stand with the feet as far apart as is comfortable.

- Point the right foot and turn the left foot in a little.

- Bend the right knee, bringing the right forearm onto the right thigh and the left hand onto the left hip.

- Rotate your pelvis back, allowing the left inner thigh to move back, lining up the outer left hip with the left ankle bone. This should pitch your upper body forward a little.

- Keeping the legs stable, try to extend the body trying to align the shoulder with the hip and ankle. This will require a lot of tone in the pelvic floor and lower abdomen. Don't allow the left thigh to move forward.

• Repeat on the second side.

TRIANGLE

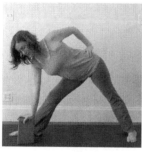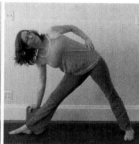

• Stand with the feet as far apart as is comfortable.

• Point the right foot and turn the left foot in 45 degrees.

• Place the right hand on a block on the outside of the right ankle, and bring the left hand to the hip.

• Rotate your pelvis back, allowing the left inner thigh to move back in space, lining up the outer left hip with the left ankle bone. This should pitch your upper body forward a little. (picture on left)

- Keeping the left hip aligned with the left ankle, try to rotate the body and stack the shoulders on top of one another. You need open hips and a strong core to keep the thighs back and lift the trunk. Keep the belly strong and the spine steady as you go.

- Repeat on the second side.

DEEP LUNGE

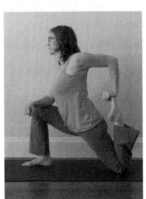

This is a very deep stretch of the psoas that shouldn't be attempted before the psoas feels long and strong and ready for more intense work.

- Starting on your hands and knees or in Downward Facing Dog, step the right foot forward.

- Place the right forearm on the right thigh.

- Bend the left leg and take hold of the left foot with the left hand.

- Draw the foot as close as possible to your left sit bone, trying to turn the pelvis and trunk to point forward.

- When you get your heel as close to the sit bone as possible, begin to move the hips forward. The right knee can go past the right ankle in the stretch.

- Try to keep the distance between the heel and the sit bone the same as you move the pelvis forward.

- Repeat on the second side.

WALL PLANK

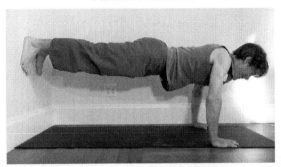

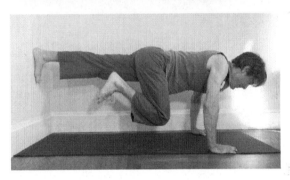

This is not easy.

- Lay prone on the floor with your feet up against the base of a wall. Bring your hands up alongside your chest.

- Straighten your arms, and walk your feet up the wall until they're level with your shoulders.

- If you are able to maintain this position, take the right foot off the wall and draw your right knee toward your chest. Maintain a stable trunk.

- Repeat with the left knee.

Chapter X

BLOG POSTS

How Do You Know If You Have A Tight Psoas?

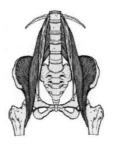

Everyone has a tight psoas, or at least one that is tighter than the other. There is no such thing as true ambidexterity. No one is perfectly balanced on both sides: handedness is part of our design. In general, we are dominant on one side though that dominance can switch top to bottom.

The question then becomes how do I know if I have a too tight psoas, or one that is causing my problems? Even though I work with back and other types of physical pain, I am not a physical therapist and don't do a lot of muscle testing.

It isn't that I find tests to be unnecessary, but they don't tend to help me help people change. If someone shows up to see me with back or any other type of pain, I take it for granted that they don't move well and start to work on changing their intrinsic patterns.

For me changing patterns is how I approach pain problems because whether you have a tight psoas or not is actually rather meaningless

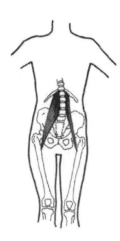

compared to how you use your psoas in daily life. I am probably being too simple (though it has served me so far) but I take it for granted that almost all back, hip and groin pain involves a tight psoas so what is the real need to test and affirm that.

That said, in all of my psoas workshops I ask people to feel for their tighter psoas to develop an understanding of their hip joint and its available rotation.

One of the standard releases that I work with called **Foot on a Block**, is one way I ask people to feel which their tight psoas is. If you stand on a block with one foot and hang the other foot off the block towards the floor, you should ideally feel which leg is more willing to release out of its socket. The leg that isn't interested in letting go is your tight psoas.

But I know from offering this thousands of times, not everybody is tuned in to this type of feeling.

From a yoga perspective I used to offer this very unscientific test for psoas length.

- Go up into a handstand at the wall with your hands as close to the wall as possible.

- Start with both heels against the wall and start to lower one leg straight down keeping the opposite heel on the wall.

- At a certain point the heel on the wall will not be able to stay connected as the lowering leg descends.

- The leg that pulls the heel off of the wall first is the tight psoas.

Don't Touch My Psoas

In my way of thinking, the psoas is the emotional muscle but what does that really mean. When I teach that we hold our emotions in our psoas—can that be literal? I don't honestly know for sure, but I don't let anyone touch my psoas.

That's just my personal preference but I think it is a good approach for most. Many years ago (before I became aware?) there was an acupuncturist who liked to needle my psoas and every time he did electric shocks would shoot out of my big toes.

One of the main phrases that I like to throw around concerning yoga is that the goal is to feel nothing. If all goes well with our practice and our muscles there is no reason to be feeling them, they are working as designed and sensation doesn't have to be part of execution.

We feel muscles when they are unhappy and the feeling of an unhappy psoas often feels different than others. It can be called the vomit muscles because that is often the feeling you get when you stretch a psoas that is not in the mood.

Not many muscles make you want to throw up when you call on them to work but the sense of nausea that often accompanies the stretching of a tight psoas is a very common reaction.

I also know of much more severe reactions that people have had, from extremely hot or cold extremities, to fever, to sleeplessness.

But not everyone is affected by having their psoas touched. At a yoga therapy training I attended about fifteen years ago I worked with someone who asked, "Do you want to touch my psoas?"

How could I resist?

With a circle of people all around us she guided me to her psoas. Then she asked me if I wanted to touch her spine from the front, which I did, though it was kind of creepy.

When I teach that we hold our emotions in our psoas—can that be literal? I don't honestly know for sure, but I don't let anyone touch my psoas.

When I teach that we hold our emotions in our psoas—can that be literal? I don't honestly know for sure, but I don't let anyone touch my psoas.

On the Level with the Psoas and the Diaphragm

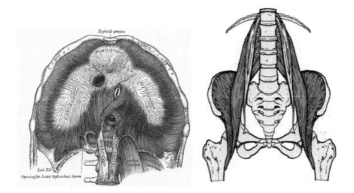

This isn't my first post about the relationship between the psoas and the diaphragm. The essential connection between the psoas and the diaphragm has a profound influence on how well our bodies function.

Considering the diaphragm as the main muscle of breathing and the psoas as the main muscle of walking, you can't take a step that doesn't involve the diaphragm or a breath that doesn't involve the psoas. And if you don't have good posture, neither the diaphragm nor the psoas will work correctly.

The iliopsoas muscle group is composed of the iliacus, psoas major and psoas minor. The iliacus and psoas major share a common tendon that attaches on the back half of the inner thigh on a knob of bone called the lesser trochanter. Sharing a common tendon means that they share certain functions.

While both the psoas major and the iliacus act as flexors of the hip the psoas major has other responsibilities as well. It is involved in external rotation of the thigh, it stabilizes the connection of the leg into the pelvis where the femoral head inserts into the acetabulum, and also assists to stabilize and erect the lower spine.

The diaphragm is the main muscle of respiration and it is different from most muscles in the body. For one, it has openings (hiatuses) that allow for structures to pass through from the upper to lower trunk. The esophagus, abdominal aorta, vena cava all traverse the diaphragm to get from the chest to the abdomen. You don't find a lot of muscles with stuff passing through them.

This is a dome like shape at the base of the ribcage its origin is at the back along the vertebrae of the spine and at the front on the ribs and the sternum. There is a central tendon that acts as an insertion point for the diaphragm muscle. When we inhale and air is pulled into the lungs, the contraction of the diaphragm pulls this central tendon down allowing for air to inflate the lungs.

While the origins and insertions that I just listed suggest two separate muscles here are a few ways the diaphragm and psoas are intricately linked. The median arcuate ligament is under the diaphragm, formed by the right and left crura of the diaphragm and passes directly over the psoas major.

The diaphragm has two crura, or tendons, that attach the diaphragm to the vertebral column. Just as the psoas major attaches along the lumbar spine, the crura of the diaphragm attach there as well. The right crus attach on the upper three lumbar vertebrae and the left crus attaches on the top two.

No muscles work in isolation and everything in the body is connected—in some ways more literally than others. A good working relationship of the psoas and the diaphragm allows them to function as designed and is integral to having a body that functions well and ages gracefully.

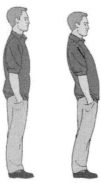

Above you'll find my two standard pictures of posture. From my perspective the good posture on the left is embodied by few, and the poor posture on the right is the default alignment for the majority of the planet.

For what it is worth, I think most people lean back like the picture on the right though most people do not perceive themselves that way (which is the subject of a few dozen blog posts).

The good posture picture on the left gives the psoas and the diaphragm a fighting chance to work together.

Two alignment features required for the harmonic convergence of the diaphragm and psoas are:

- The legs must be directly under the pelvis so the psoas can successfully stabilize the connection of the leg to the pelvis.

- The base of the pelvis, ribcage and floor need to be parallel to each other.

Setting the leg correctly into the hip socket and leveling the base of the rib cage allows these tacitly connected muscles to work as a unit or team driving the body to heights of functional efficiency.

The Role of the Psoas in Walking

You would be hard pressed to find someone to tell you that walking isn't good exercise. There aren't many givens in our world but this is one of them—walking is good for you.

What is interesting about these general pronouncements is they never, and I mean never, talk about how you should walk.

The psoas major is my favorite muscle, the body's most important muscle and the main engine of walking. And my pronouncement today is walking is only good for you if you use the psoas correctly.

Three muscles connect the legs to the spine (psoas, piriformis and gluteus maximus) but only the psoas connects from the front of the body and to the lumbar spine. In fact the psoas created the curve in the lumbar spine when we began to walk upright, and its connection to this section of the body is what makes it so important.

If the skeleton is well aligned which means the leg bones, or femurs, are directly under the pelvis, the psoas can initiate each step from the deep core. What this looks like when walking is a foot that falls under the knee and relatively close to the pelvis, equidistant from the opposite leg.

The question then is what initiates the step if not the psoas? What usually happens is the legs move forward too far and too fast which leaves the quadriceps (thigh) and adductor (inner thighs) muscles to begin the journey of ambulation.

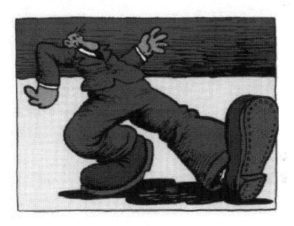

When walking is going well every step is a spinal twist that not only moves the body but stimulates, lubricates and tones it. The body that moves well is a self-healing machine and that healing only happens with a functional psoas.

When we are walking well with the good use of the psoas, the pelvis tilts and rotates in such a way as to create the above mentioned spinal twist. When we fail to use the psoas and walk correctly the pelvis tends to get stuck and hike up from side to side rather than tilt and rotate.

This very common pattern eliminates so many of the possible benefits derived from walking correctly with the psoas.

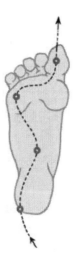

Steps that are initiated with the quadriceps and adductors tend to move through the outside of the foot which minimizes the ability of the psoas to help with walking. Every step we take ends with the inner foot on the mound of the big toe.

The big toe corresponds to the inner upper thigh and the psoas. When a step is completed successfully the psoas of the back leg is activated through this inner foot/inner thigh connection.

This successful movement through the back leg stabilizes that side of the body and spine as the opposite leg and psoas is released to come forward.

There is very little in our musculature that is not involved with good walking technique. The psoas major, iliacus, all four pairs of abdominal muscles, erector spinea, IT Band, and so on, up and down the chain of good movement.

The Psoas, Erector Spinae and Lower Back Pain

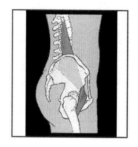

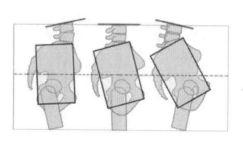 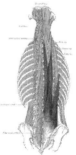

The big pronouncement of today's post is that it is hard to resolve lower back pain if the femurs, or leg bones, don't sit directly under the pelvis (as in the middle image of the middle image above).

Making this bony alignment happen is the magic ingredient for the relief of lower back pain. Lower back pain can happen for many reasons and sometimes there are structural problems that we have very little control over.

We can be born with, or inherit spinal issues, that occur before we are even aware of our own movements. Other times accidents, injuries or even illness can create an environment that leads to pain and dysfunction.

But I have found that poor posture is the cause of a great deal of back pain. Back pain is so common and so diverse in its origin and manifestation that its causes and effects can never really be lumped into one easy package but posture can cover a wide range of back problems.

We will consider my favorite muscle — the psoas — and how its poor alignment can render the erector spinae muscles, that are meant to extend our spine, useless.

The curve in our lower spine is what allows us to be upright and walk on two legs. This curve, when functional, facilitates the transfer of weight from the head down to the pelvis and legs.

The curve in our lower spine, created by the psoas when we began to stand and walk upright on two legs, is needed for the erector spinae muscles to do their job and extend the spine upwards.

The erector muscles, work in a chain up and down the spine. All links in the chain need to be aligned for the chain to work well. This can only work well if the legs, pelvis and lower back are aligned so that the psoas when properly placed, allows access for the extension of the vertebral column. This happens when the femur bone sits directly under the center of the lumbar spine.

I have written previously about this in so many contexts but when the legs pelvis and lumbar spine are correctly situated the psoas can work like a pulley to allow for the full extension of the spine.

If the legs sink forward of the pelvis as they so often do, the psoas loses the tension created when is crosses the rim of the pelvis to align under the back half of the body.

If the psoas aligns correctly the lumbar vertebrae are pulled forward and down and they can find optimal length and spacing in a gentle curve which frees the erector spinae muscles to extend the spine as designed.

The end result is a more spacious lower back because the good alignment of the skeleton allow the muscles that are meant to extend the spine to do their job as designed.

The Psoas and Quadratus Lumborum

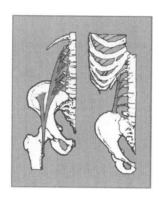

When it comes to the psoas and quadratus lumborum, you can't have problems in one without having trouble with the other.

They are two muscles with completely different functions yet they connect to the spine in a similar fashion which leaves them inextricably related.

The quadratus lumborum as its name implies is a quadrate muscle which means that it acts as a stabilizer–in this case stabilizing the pelvis to the ribcage. It functions mainly is as a side bending muscle.

The psoas is a hip flexor that also externally rotates the thigh. It also lifts the trunk off of the floor from a supine position. In addition, the spine stack vertically above the pelvis with the essential aid of the psoas, and it is also the most important muscle in a successful gait pattern.

Looking at the image above it is fairly easy to see–since they attach to almost the exact same places on the spine– why the tone in one of these two muscles so profoundly affects the other.

What goes for the psoas and quadratus lumborum goes for all of the muscles in what I'll refer to as the pelvic belt.

The quadratus lumborum is like a bed sheet pinned along three sides and spread out evenly. When the psoas is tight that right side of the Ql can no longer expand as much as the left and you have a lopsided rectangle.

At that point you can hardly blame the quadratus lumborum for failing to function well.

Is the Psoas Always a Factor in Lower Back Pain?

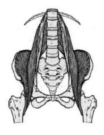

While the psoas muscle might not be the cause of all of your lower back pain it is invariably involved in some way or another in pretty much every incidence of lumbar spine and lower back problems.

As the psoas is the only muscle connecting the legs to the spine above the pelvis it would be difficult for this not to be the case.

I often return to the idea that the psoas is the body's most important muscle for three reasons.

- The psoas muscle helps us stand upright which is kind of key to being human.

- It walks us through life as the muscle that initiates each successful step we take.

- It gets interesting when we consider the psoas to be the warehouse of the body's unprocessed energy and trauma.

All three of these concepts revolve around the lumbar spine along which the psoas attaches, and actually creates when we first stand and begin to walk upright.

If the spine suffers the psoas suffers so it doesn't matter which of the following issues someone might be dealing with, the psoas will be affected.

Here are some more bullets covering some spine and disc issues, though back pain isn't exclusive to this club:

- Stenosis
- Herniation's
- Spondylosis
- Spondylolysis
- Spondylolisthesis

The psoas attaches at six points—one below the pelvis and five above.

Below the pelvis, the psoas inserts with the iliacus, as they form a common tendon, onto the lesser trochanter at the back of the femur bone.

Above, the psoas originates from the bodies and the bases of the transverse processes of the 12th thoracic vertebrae through the fourth lumbar vertebrae (T12-L4).

The bones of the lumbar spine are meant to stack one on top of the other. They are big fat bones that bear weight and allow for very little rotational movement.

Any of the above conditions— and there are others that could be added to the list— will mess with the ideal alignment of the bones which will throw off the ideal alignment of the psoas.

A well-aligned psoas supports the lift and extension of the entire spine. A well-aligned psoas can limit the chances of these types of degenerative issues occurring or worsening.

But unfortunately the reverse is true as well. As disks degenerate for whatever reason their movement or calcification can disable the psoas ability to function fully and efficiently as the attachment at each of the vertebrae influences the others.

My recipe for supporting these issues has four ingredients so here are some more bullets:

- Release your psoas

- Improve your posture

- Develop balanced core tone

- Find better movement patterns

The Pelvis, the Psoas and the Masseter Muscle

The masseter muscle connects the jaw to the skull. If your jaw aches, odds are the masseter is involved. Likewise, the masseter is by nature involved when people suffer from jaw dysfunction, commonly referred to as TMD, or TMJD. It isn't the only muscle in the mix so you will be feeling all the involved muscles of the jaw in the following exercise.

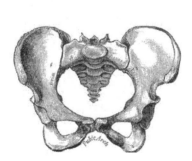
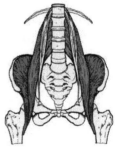

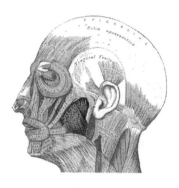

The alignment of the pelvis (and the legs underneath the pelvis), determines in large part the alignment of the psoas. Together these two partners when we'll situated, facilitate ease in the body both postural and emotionally.

Well situated for me means that the leg bones fall directly underneath the hips and your big butt muscle gluteus maximus doesn't sit on the hamstring. It should have a room of its own, so to speak, and that is one way to know that your pelvis is in a good neutral position.

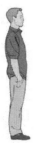 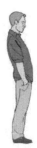

The psoas is in a good position when the bottom of it, where it attaches to the back of the femur bone, is aligned with the back half of the body.

The opposite, where I think most people spend the majority of their time, is for the thigh bones to sink or lean forward which forces the gluteus maximus to sit down on the back of the thigh or hamstrings. This also moves the attachment of the psoas to the front half of the body.

For the following exercise I want you to switch back and forth between these two positions. Feel free to go to extremes in both directions. The point is to feel the muscles of the jaw and how they respond to the different ways the bones align when you shift the pelvis from tucked under to stuck out.

I think that there is a correct or best alignment of the pelvis and psoas. I believe that you know that you are there when the majority of your muscles relax when not in a state of action. In this case we are feeling the masseter and muscles of the jaw.

This is an experiential exercise that is very easy to tap into, and very easy to do, and hopefully, allows you to tap into the functioning of your muscles.

Feel the Masseter and the Jaw

- Stand with the feet as close together as comfortable.

- If it is comfortable, close your eyes.

- Start by standing in a position that you consider good posture.

- Bring your awareness to your jaw. How does it hang? Do the muscles feel tight? Loose? Etc.

- Now lean the thighs forward and tuck the pelvis under keeping your awareness on the jaw and how changing your posture changes your jaw.

- Then stick your butt out and take the thighs back (though you can do this in any order that you'd like).

- Move back and forth this way feeling the changes in tone to the jaw and its assorted connective tissue.

- Find the placement of the pelvis where the jaw and masseter muscles feel best.

If I had to guess the legs will be under the hips, the gluteus maximus will have a room of its own and your psoas will be set back at is base so that it can perform its magic.

The Psoas, Forward Head Posture and the Scalene Muscles

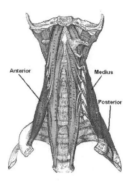

The scalene muscles are three paired muscles of differing lengths. They originate from the transverse process of the 2nd-7th cervical vertebrae (the neck), and insert on the first and second ribs.

They are three (sometimes four) muscles that act to flex, bend and rotate the neck depending on how they are working together and what part of the skeleton is fixed or moving. If the ribcage doesn't move, all three of the scalene muscles can bend the neck forward and sideways, and rotate it as well.

When the head and neck are held steady, the scalenus anterior and medius both elevate the first rib while the scalenus posterior elevates the second rib to assist in breathing and create more space in the thoracic cavity.

Forward head posture is endemic to our society. If you live and breathe the odds are you suffer from this postural problem. And if you do, the scalene muscles are part of the problem. Take some pictures of yourself, look in a mirror or try to stand with your back to the wall and get the entire back of your body (other than the lower back and the neck) to the wall. If your head doesn't get there comfortably you have tight scalene muscles and forward head posture.

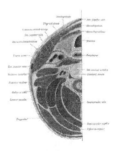

I can promise that you are not alone.

Forward head posture creates an imbalance between the muscles of the head neck and shoulders. The muscles in front of your neck tend to become over-extended while those at the back of the neck usually are short, tight and suffering.

When the scalenes and sternocleidomastoid (SCM) are pulled forward posturally, the erector spinea muscles, meant to elevate the spine are pulled forward as well, and lose their erectile capabilities.

Another part of the head and neck that is affected are the sub occipital muscles connecting the head to the top of the spine. These are the only muscles in the body with a connection to the spinal cord, and their ability to communicate with the spine is severely compromised by forward head posture and misaligned scalene muscles.

Most pains in the neck involve the scalene muscles to one degree or another. You can suffer from tight scalenes on one side of the neck as well. A dysfunctional psoas major (my favorite muscle) often creates a leg length discrepancy which can inhibit or shorten the entire side of the body, including and creating short tight scalenes.

The scalene muscles, along with the SCM are situated in a key spot in our anatomical structure and therefore can be involved with numerous nerve pain related problems. The nerves need space to flow in order to power the body and tight muscles often mess with the optimal flow of nervous energy.

The most critical aspect of misaligned scalene muscles occurs with the brachial plexus, a network of nerves that emanate from the spine, passing through the neck, on the way to innervate the arm. The brachial plexus' route from the spine to the arm passes directly between scalenus anterior and scalenus medius. Short, tight or generally misaligned scalene muscles can impact the brachial plexus directly.

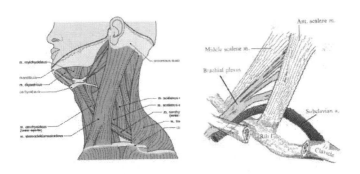

The list of problems that can be related to the brachial plexus is fairly long and while the scalene muscles might not be the exact cause they will always be related to head neck and shoulder issues of forward head posture. Carpal tunnel syndrome, thoracic outlet syndrome, numb extremities are just a few options on a long menu of ailments.

The most effective way to bring relief to unhappy scalenes is to change the posture that led to their suffering in the first place. Finding this relief will not come from moving the head and neck, but by reorienting the pelvis so that it frees the spine to stack vertically and allows the head to sit comfortably on top of the vertebral column.

A well aligned spine with a free and happy psoas affords the body the best chance to work according to its design. Its design is pretty magical but it is not fulfilled through osmosis. We need to think about the way we walk and stand if we want our heads to sit on straight on our scalene muscles to be successfully aligned.

The Psoas, the Lumbar Spine and Lower Back Pain

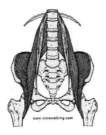

The psoas major muscle attaches along the lumbar spine and lower back pain often involves this all-important muscle that too few people have heard of. The five bones that make up the lumbar spine sit between the pelvis and the rib cage, bearing and transferring weight from the upper to lower body.

The psoas flexes and laterally rotates the leg at the hip and it flexes the spine. From a standing position the psoas lifts the leg bending the knee towards the chest. Lying on the floor the psoas helps to lift the trunk towards a sit up.

The curve of the lumbar spine, without which we couldn't stand or walk upright, is created by the psoas major when we stand up from a kneeling and crawling position. When the psoas shortens or engages it pulls the lumbar vertebrae forward and down. This engagement is what created our curved lower spine as the pelvis is pulled upright with the spine stacked vertically.

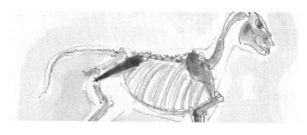

The lower back in a quadrupedal animal lacks a curve because the psoas doesn't cross the pelvis to affect the lumbar spine.

When it comes to the lumbar spine and lower back pain it is hard, if not impossible, for the psoas muscle to avoid complicity in the problem at hand. The same goes for many of the muscles in the vicinity of the psoas.

The quadratus lumborum, for example, is the next door neighbor of the psoas, connecting the pelvis to the ribcage and acting to stabilize these structures. The quadratus, or QL, attaches to similar points along the lumbar spine as the psoas and they are almost always part of the lower back pain puzzle.

The psoas can affect the lumbar spine in many ways as it connects to four of the lumbar vertebrae in two different places (both the body and the base of the transverse processes).

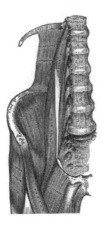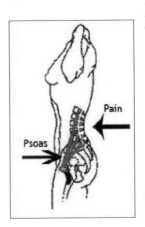

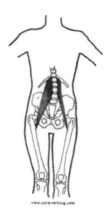

If the engaged psoas pulls the lumbar vertebrae forward, chronically tight psoas muscles will
pull and keep the lumbar vertebrae forward into a
hyper lordotic, or overly arched, state. If the psoas
is tight on only one side it will pull the vertebrae
forward on that side only and in turn will usually
twist and torque the pelvis along with the lum-
bars. As one side tightens, the other side often
fades into obscurity losing tone and strength.

Both of these inappropriate alignments of the
psoas can, and often do, lead to lower back pain.
These are basic misalignments that involve all of
the connections of the psoas along the lumbar
spine. But it is also possible for the psoas to have

problems within the individual connections along the spine.

If the psoas attaches on the first through fourth lumbar vertebrae it is possible for two of those attachments to be happily aligned and two to be off kilter.

With all of these possibilities for dysfunction there are many ways to connect the psoas, the lumbar spine and lower back pain. Too tight psoas can compress the lumbar vertebrae creating pain in the center of the spine. One tight psoas can compress the spine laterally creating lower back pain that would present slightly different symptoms.

One tight psoas can also pull a leg up into the hip socket limiting range of motion and creating discomfort. That same tight psoas can push forward into the inguinal ligament creating yet another kind of pain that often presents as a wrapping feeling from the front of the pelvis towards the back.

The psoas, the lumbar spine and lower back pain are usually synonymous in my book. And even if the psoas isn't directly involved with the pain, getting the psoas aligned and working more functionally is almost always part of the healing puzzle.

The Psoas Major and Rectus Femoris

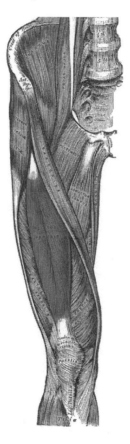

The psoas major and rectus femoris both flex the hip. Additionally, the psoas externally rotates the leg and rectus femoris extends the leg at the knee. As with so many of the surrounding muscles it is hard to have problems with the psoas major that don't also involve the rectus femoris and vice versa.

These two muscles might suffer more from poor posture than any other in the body due to their proximity to the temple of postural confusion that is the pelvis.

Good posture means that our bones are aligned in a way that allows them to stack one upon the other in a fashion that allows weight to transfer through the bones. When the bones are aligned in this way the muscles have an opportunity to live in balanced harmony.

When the bones are misaligned the muscles will suffer because they will have to pick up the supportive slack created by the off kilter bones.

The pelvis is like the hub of a wheel. If it is off center the whole wheel will suffer and it won't be able to turn efficiently. The same goes for the pelvis and the body's posture. The alignment of the pelvis determines everything that happens above and below it. The slightest deviation from neutral will negatively affect everything that emanates from the pelvis.

The psoas major is one of only three muscles that connect the legs to the spine and the only one that does so from the front of the body. The rectus femoris is the only one of the four quadriceps muscles that connects to the pelvis. These two muscles are the main flexors of the hip and have a hard time functioning successfully when the pelvis is improperly aligned.

There are two main postural problems with the pelvis.

1. Most people are living with their pelvis tucked under, or tilted posteriorly.

2. The legs usually fail to line up underneath the pelvis. They usually lean slightly forward which pulls on the pelvis, often towards a posterior tilt.

When these two issues occur, both the psoas major and rectus femoris are pushed out of their comfort zone and natural resting place. The forward thrust of the legs and the pelvis put undue strain on the rectus femoris actually asking it bear quite a bit of weight from the upper body which is not at all its job.

In the case of the psoas, the forward leaning legs, which take the pubic bone along for the ride, push or pull the psoas major forward affecting the lumbar spine negatively increasing its curve in the process.

This all leads to problems for our bodies. Luckily the fix is simple, align the bones and free the muscles. That is one of our main goals as we go through this book.

The Big Toe, the Psoas and Lower Back Pain

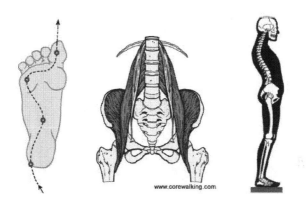

www.corewalking.com

Lower back pain can often, though not always, be traced to an issue with the psoas muscle. The psoas—the body's most important muscle—helps to hold the spine upright, facilitates good walking patterns and warehouses all of the body's unprocessed energy.

The relationship of the psoas to lower back pain encompasses all three of these factors. Our unprocessed energy can lead to back pain for esoteric reasons that are unrelated to the big toe, but we will cover that information later.

But when it comes to walking and standing the big toe is easily connected to incidents of lower back pain as related to the psoas. Much of this pain can be attributed to a lack of support for the lumbar spine due to the misalignment of the pelvis, legs and in turn, the psoas.

The psoas attaches on the femur bone towards the back of the inner thigh. It is essential for the psoas to align in the back plane of the body at its top and bottom if it is to successfully hold the spine upright and initiate our gait. To do so the legs need to sit directly under the hips.

When we put weight onto the big toe and the inner edge of the foot we activate the inner thigh at the same time. When we walk correctly the entire weight of the body falls on the big toe in order to push off to the next step. Pushing off through the big toe activates the inner thighs and sets the psoas back at its base.

This action also helps the spine to lengthen. When the inner thigh moves backwards, taking the psoas with it, the psoas engages across the rim of the pelvis pulling the lumbar spine forward. The erector muscles of the spine react to the shortening of the psoas by moving in opposition and extending up the back of the body.

The easiest way to feel the connection between the psoas and the big toe is to stand up with the feet parallel and hip distance apart.

- Roll your weight onto the outside of your feet and you will likely feel the outer thighs engage and your inner thighs lose tone.

- Roll onto the inner edge of the foot particularly the mound of the big toe and feel the inner thighs tone slightly.

The power of this weight shift should not be underestimated. It is this grounding, or lack thereof, that can be responsible for a great deal of lower back pain. When we bear the weight of the upper body through the outer foot we lose access to our center and to the psoas muscle.

A great deal of the lower back pain that people experience comes from faulty load bearing and compression of the lumbar vertebrae due to poor posture and weight transfer.

If the psoas isn't properly aligned at the back half of the inner thigh with the legs directly under the pelvis and the inner foot bearing its share of the load, the psoas can't work in tandem with spinal erectors and the lower spine will be compressed which in many cases can lead to lower back pain.

The Pelvis, The Psoas And That Tight Pectoralis Minor

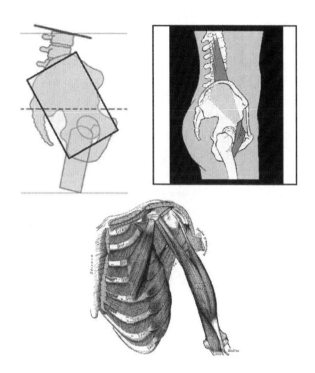

Tight pectoralis minor muscles are a problem for a large majority of people that I work with. Pectoralis minorconnects the shoulder girdle to the rib cage and functions to draw the shoulder blade forward and down. It tends to become tight and dysfunctional for a number of reasons.

It would be easy to blame the computer that you hunch over for hours on end as the main culprit, or the vegetables you chop, or the baby you carry... these actions all make it easy to develop a tight pectoralis minor.

But, and there is always the inevitable but, if your pelvis and lumbar curve are correctly aligned you should have adequate support for these functionally necessary postural positions.

When you sit or stand with the pelvis tucked under, or the thighs leaning forward, it throws off the natural curve of the lumbar spine which profoundly influences the pectoralis minor and its partner pectoralis major.

I have written previously about the relationship of the alignment of the pelvis and the rhomboid muscles of the upper back and this pretty much means the same territory.

When the pelvis is in the right place, the psoas muscles help the erector muscles of the spine to lengthen, providing support for the usually loose rhomboids to tone.

The same thing happens to the tight pectoralis

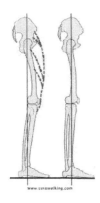

www.curawalking.com

minor muscle. The extension of the spine facilitated by the pelvis and psoas broadens pectoralis minor. It might resist that broadening in a different way than the looser more lax rhomboid but with persistence and the right stretches, the tight pectoralis minor muscle will eventually begin to open.

But, and there often is another but, all the body work and upper body stretching in the world won't address the issue of a tight pectoralis minor if you don't change your posture and realign the lower body as well.

If you learn to walk and stand correctly, the pectoral muscles with have a much better chance to align and open.

Scoliosis and the Psoas: Curvature of the Spine

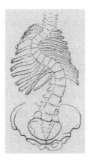

Scoliosis, the term used to describe an excessive curvature of the spine, may have its genesis in a tight psoas muscle. Everyone is dominant on one side of the body and it is not likely that any body's spine is completely straight, but the term scoliosis is applied when the curvature of the spine is greater than 10 degrees.

Scoliosis can occur at a number of times during someone's life. Sometimes the curvature of the spine can be congenital and the condition presents itself at birth. There are certain conditions that are often coupled with scoliosis such as spina bifida or cerebral palsy.

Most often the exact cause is not known and

the excessive curvature presents itself anywhere from infancy to adolescence to adulthood. In these cases I have no problem ascribing a neuromuscular issue to the curvature in the spine which is where the psoas comes in.

The psoas muscle connects the legs to the lower spine and the classic indicators of a tight psoas are often similar to the way that the curvature of the spine is diagnosed—one shoulder higher or lower than the other; one hip higher or lower than the other; and leg length discrepancy.

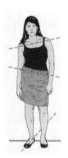

A tight psoas can seriously mess with the spine and pelvis. If the portion of the psoas that attaches to the leg is tight it can increase the curve of the lumbar spine. If the upper end of the psoas is tight it can decrease the curve.

The body always compensates in some way for muscular imbalances. If one side of the body is tight and not working all that effectively, the other side with often work harder to make up. This can effectively pull the spine in two directions.

The curvature of the spine can take on many patterns. The tight psoas can pull the lumbar vertebrae forward on one side which can begin the curving process. Anytime the spine is pulled in one direction there will be compensating forces moving in another direction.

Invariably the rib cage with get involved and depending upon the circumstances the entire spine up through the neck can get twisted in the scoliotic journey.

The Painful Relationship of the Psoas and Rectus Femoris

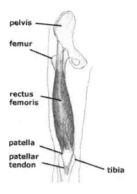

The psoas major and rectus femoris are two of the body main hip flexors (sartorius is the other).

The Psoas Major

The psoas major is the most important muscle in the body. It walks us forward through life, it warehouses all of our unprocessed emotions and it is goes a long way to keep the spine upright on top of the pelvis. The psoas at the front and the gluteus maximus and piriformis in the back are connecting the legs to the pelvis, and between them, holding the spine aloft if the psoas is well aligned and functioning as designed.

The Rectus Femoris

The rectus femoris is one of the four quadriceps muscles. The four quadriceps muscles all meet to insert into the tibia of the shin. But the rectus femoris is the only one of these muscles that connects to the pelvis. The others—vastus lateralis, medialis and intermedius—all connect to the femur or thigh bone. The quadriceps is essentially an extensor of the knee, and only the rectus femoris plays a role in hip flexion.

I am obsessed with getting people to <u>stop</u> tucking the pelvis. The other piece to untucking is getting the thighs to move directly under the hips. This thigh alignment is key to getting the psoas to work as it is designed and the for the rectus femoris to work successfully as a hip flexor.

The psoas acts like a pulley system in the body. A pulley is a simple machine and viewed from the side, the hip bone is the pulley and the psoas is the rope. The pulley work of the psoas facilitates the reciprocal inhibition that allows the extensor muscles of the spine to lengthen.

The psoas can only act like a pulley if the legs are under the hips. If the legs are where they should be, the psoas moves down from its origin at the base of the rib cage/top of the lumbar spine, to move forward crossing the rim of the pelvis, and then moves back again to insert on the lesser trochanter a knob of bone on the back half of the thigh.

It is the back/ front/back arrangement that foster the psoas ability to help support the spine on top of the pelvis. For this to happen the thighs have to be under the hips. When the pelvis tucks under and the thighs move forward taking the psoas with them, the tension across the rim of the pelvis is lost and much of the psoas support capabilities go with it.

When the thighs go forward a great deal of stress and pressure is put on the rectus femoris muscle basically pushing it forward. When this happens the rectus femoris is called upon to support the upper body because the power of the psoas is taken out of the picture.

The Rectus Femoris Tendon

The rectus femoris tendon is really what bears the brunt of this powerful misalignment and rears its ugly head for many people when they try to do core work while lying on the back. This tendon when it is over stretched and overburdened from the weight of the upper body sinking into it tends to scream out in pain.

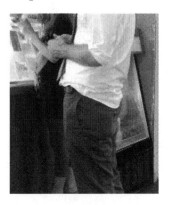

This happens literally as the tendon can pop like a steel cable and pretty much shut down all attempts to either engage the quadriceps or work in concert with the psoas. This happens most often in poses like navasana or one of my key exercises feet three inches off the floor.

This has all been another reminderto stop tucking your pelvis and start getting your thighs to move under your hips. The effort will pay off in a big way.

Treatment for Psoas Pain

Psoas pain can take a lot of different forms and finding treatment for it is often mysterious and elusive. I can't tell you the number of clients who come my way after suffering years of pain without anyone telling them exactly what is wrong with their body.

Treatment for pain that is not identifiable in ordinary measures is not going to be easy to find through traditional means. Psoas pain is often limited to the lower back. But just as often it manifests in a wrapping pain from the groin to the top of the pelvis and back. Sometimes it shows as groin pain and sometimes as outer hip discomfort. Psoas pain is occasionally stable and localized but just as often it hurts in one place in the morning and shifts to another area in the afternoon.

Many people who suffer from psoas pain go to doctors who send them for x-rays and MRI's only to be told that there is nothing wrong as far as the machines can see.

People referred to physical therapy for the treatment of psoas pain, even if correctly diagnosed, are often given a standard protocol of stretches that in my mind don't often do much to get to the heart of the problem. Psoas stretches are great but they aren't often the answer for psoas related pain.

Treatment for Psoas Pain

Treatment for psoas pain falls into two categories for me—releasing the psoas, and learning to walk correctly as a means to change long held movement patterns that either led to the problem or exacerbated it.

Stretching the psoas has it place only after successfully releasing it. There are a whole host of psoas releases that I work with though it is a good bet to start with Constructive Rest Position which I have written about earlier in the book.

The psoas is the main muscle of walking so spending time learning how to walk correctly— and I meet very few people who walk correctly– is the best treatment for psoas pain. Walking with a psoas that is employed successfully along with the right release exercises can go a long way to alleviate all sorts of lower back, hip, groin and knee pain.

Psoas And Iliacus Stretch:
Handstand Split

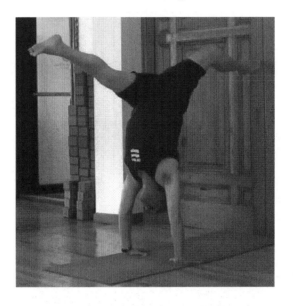

The following psoas and iliacus stretch is part of that eBook and definitely falls under advanced. Hanumanasana or forward split has been my favorite yoga pose since the day I started practicing.

I have unusually long hamstrings and equally open hips, so I was basically born to do this stretch.

The <u>psoas</u> and iliacus together are called the

iliopsoas because they meet and form a common tendon that connects to a knob of bone called the lesser trochanter. The iliacus goes from the lesser trochanter to wrap the inside of the hip or bowl of the pelvis, while the psoas rises up to attach along the lumbar spine.

Almost every psoas stretch is also an ilacus stretch because of their mutual attachment at the inner thigh. Along with my loose hamstrings I have very long psoas muscles and don't often feel the psoas and iliacus when doing conventional stretches of these muscles.

But when I do a handstand and work my split while upside down I can get an extremely sensational stretch of both the psoas and iliacus muscles. The key to getting the deepest stretch in this position is to square the hips as much as you can while separating the legs as far apart as possible, as well as engaging the abdominals to the best of your ability.

There are two important factors to be aware of.

1. If you usually work near the wall for your handstand practice it can be scary to move so far into the middle of the room and trust that the wall will catch you.

2. It can be hard to feel where the legs are when you are upside down and it might take a number of attempts before you can either get the legs to fully separate or get the feet to lower to similar levels. The foot on the wall tends to be lower than the foot towards the middle of the room.

Psoas and Iliacus Stretch: Handstand Split

- You can eyeball the distance that the hand should be from the wall or set up with your hands a legs length away.

- Starting from downward dog lightly kick up and bring one leg to the wall. This is the scary part and you have to trust that your leg will touch the wall and you won't collapse in a heap.

- Once one foot is on the wall extend the other

leg towards the middle of the room. Try to is often hard to feel when you are upside down.

- The psoas stretch comes in the squaring of the hips. It is always easier to let the hips turn open. Keep trying to turn the pelvis so that the outer hips are on the same plane. The more you can do this and engage the abdominals the more the psoas will stretch.

The Psoas Muscle Created the Lumbar Curve

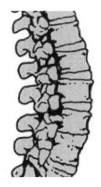 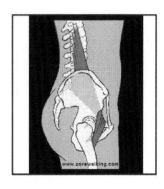

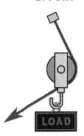

EFFORT

LOAD

The essence of the upright body lies in the lumbar curve of the spine. These five bones that have an anterior curve (inward) hold up the trunk transferring the weight of the head and shoulder to the pelvis and legs.

Without the lumbar curve we would not be able to walk upright on two legs. Our nearest relatives the chimpanzee can walk upright for a few steps before returning to their knuckles mainly because they have no lumbar curve in their spine.

In my home we have a dog and two cats who have flat lower spines because a four legged animal has no need for the lumbar curve because it has no need to remain upright any longer than it takes to lick my face or destroy our furniture with their claws.

There are numerous theories about how and why we became upright but one thing is for sure— we are the first and only mammals with a lumbar curve.

The psoas, my favorite muscle, is also known as the tenderloin. This is because in a four legged animal the psoas muscle crosses from the leg to the spine without touching the pelvis. The human psoas wouldn't be all that tender because it crosses the rim of the pelvis in a very different way than in a quadruped.

Two major changes took place when we began to stand. For one, we developed large gluteus maximus muscles. If you think of dogs, cats, horses or cows etc., they don't have our bubble-like butts. And the second development was the birth of the lumbar curve created as the psoas moved across the rim of the pelvis.

When the psoas came into contact with the pelvis tension was created as the spine moved upright on top of the legs. The tension resulted in the psoas pulling the lower spine forward bringing the lumbar curve into being.

This was a major event because it is the lumbar curve along with our thinking brain, among other traits, that makes us distinctly human.

As brilliant and astounding as this development was, the repercussions are still being dealt with and not all that successfully. As nice as it is to stand, walk, talk and do yoga, the overwhelming amount of back shoulder hip and every other pain comes from a skewed relationship that most of us have with our lumbar curve. All the work in my CoreWalking program begins with aligning the pelvis and lumbar curve and poor sitting and standing posture is almost always related to the lumbar curve being improperly aligned.

Sub Occipital Muscles, a Tucked Pelvis and the Psoas

The sub occipital muscles are directly affected by a tucked pelvis. In truth there is a much more literal connection between the psoas and the rhomboids, and the relationship that they have connecting the legs and shoulder girdle to the spine, but the sub occipital muscles are likewise affected by a tucked pelvis.

The psoas works as a pulley system within the body. One of its essential functions is to provide support to the uplifting spine. It does this pretty much any time there is a successful arch in the lumbar (lower) spine. The spine has four curves in order to successfully transfer weight from the head to the legs. If the spine were straight instead of curved it would be impossible to support the very heavy weight of the head on top of the shoulders and the pelvis.

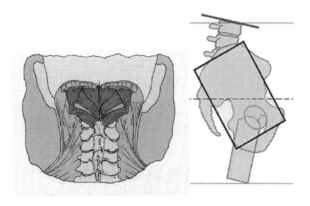

The lumbar spine is most responsible for bearing and transferring this weight. That is why the five bones of the lumbar spine are bigger than the rest of the vertebrae, and though they can flex and extend, they can't rotate. Their size and stability are designed for carrying the load of the upper body.

The four sub occipital muscles connect the head to the very top of the spine—the first two vertebrae (C1 & C2), the atlas and the axis—extend, rotate and tilt the head. But they can only really accomplish these functions if the head sits directly on top of the spine. When the head is forced forward these muscles are basically holding on for dear life which is why they very often become full of tension that can lead to profound discomfort.

The effect of the psoas and a tucked pelvis on the support of the head and sub occipital muscles is one of the easiest things to feel. Assuming that you are sitting as you read this (and I hate to say it but I am assuming that you are sitting badly, though I hope I am wrong), deepen your groins, sticking the butt out a little, bringing a small arch into the lower back. This basic action should support the head bringing it slightly back in space without your needing to do anything else.

Now tuck the pelvis rounding the lower back slightly and feel what happens to the head. If I had to guess it moved forward as the upper back rounded a bit. A tucked pelvis eliminates the lumbar curve which removes the spinal support for the head forcing it forward into space.

Sitting standing and walking correctly are essential to having a head situated happily in space, and sub occipital muscles that can work according to their design. Developing support for your head by properly aligning a tucked pelvis and activating the pulley system of the psoas can have far reaching effects that can alleviate sinus problems, headaches and chronic neck and shoulder strain.

Rhomboid Muscles, a Tucked Pelvis and the Psoas

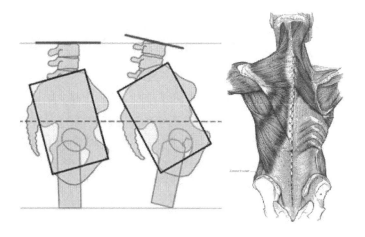

The Rhomboid muscles connect the shoulder blade to the spine at the back. The psoas major connects the spine to the legs from the front. If your pelvis is properly aligned (untucked), the psoas works like a pulley system to help lengthen and extend the spine. The pulley system works because the psoas attaches at the back of the body and crosses the front of the pelvis creating the tension that helps to support the spine. The hip bone is the pulley and the psoas is the rope.

When the psoas works as a pulley the erector

spinea muscles at the back of the body lengthen the spine upwards. If your pelvis is tucked under the bottom of the psoas moves forward and the tension that creates the pulley action disappears. What does this have to do with the rhomboid muscles you ask? Tuck your pelvis under and see for yourself. The ideal position of the shoulder blades finds them equidistant from the spine and parallel to each other at their upper border.

When the pelvis tucks under and the psoas can no longer assist the erector muscles of the spine to extend up, the shoulder blades are pulled apart and the rhomboid muscles are pulled wider apart than they need to be. This is the environment that I find most people live in—rhomboid muscles that are too long and tend towards weakness. This is a direct result of the position of the pelvis and lack of pulley action in the psoas.

I find that many people are trying to figure out their posture by taking their shoulders backwards instead of realigning the pelvis. For me taking the shoulders back creates a false sense of good posture because it creates tone in the rhomboid muscles that can't be sustained if the pelvis is misaligned.

The two things that need to happen are untucking the pelvis which allows the psoas to do its thing and creates a better more natural placement of the shoulder blades, and, building tone in the rhomboids through exercises. If these things happen no one will need to hold their shoulders and arms up and back because they will be naturally aligned.

Posture needs to develop from the placement of the pelvis, not be created by taking the arms and shoulders, and in turn the rhomboid muscles, where we think they should be. Posture should be the natural result of good skeletal alignment and balanced muscle tone. Not something we are actively creating by holding ourselves in place.

The Psoas Major and the Transverse Abdominis Muscle

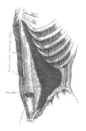

The transverse abdominis muscle and the psoas major are intimately connected in the exercise, Feet Three Inches off the Floor (don't you love the catchy title?) that is in the stretching section in the middle of this book. This exercise is one of the Core Four exercises that I assign at the outset of my CoreWalking Program.

The transverse abdominis muscle is a deep abdominal muscle that helps to stabilize the spine in this essential exercise. The spine is a magical piece of equipment usually made up of 26 bones with four curves. The psoas major is the muscle that holds us up, walks us through life and warehouses our trauma and unprocessed energy (pretty big stuff).

They all interact in the exercise Feet Three Inches off the floor. As a collection of bone the spine is highly mobile. It bends, twists, extends and flexes. But it also solidifies. This dynamic of supple and solid is at the root of what I am trying to teach in my yoga classes. Ideally the spine should be highly mobile at times—for positions such as cat and cow—and a rigid pole at other times—such as plank.

There are different issues when it comes to the mobility of the spine, or the lack thereof. Some people are too loose in both the ligaments and muscles, while some are too tight. An immobile spine is not easy to figure out. As loose as I am in most of my joints, before I did an extensive course of treatment with a chiropractor about seven or eight years ago, my lumbar spine (lower back) did not move. And it took about six months of regular treatments before it gained the fluidity it has maintained ever since.

When working on the exercise Feet Three Inches Off The Floor, the psoas major does the work to lift the feet up. I always start with one foot at a time to be nice to the psoas, hip flexors and pelvis. This lifting of the foot by the psoas major is one of its essential functions but not the point of the pose.

This pose explores and develops the tone in the transverse abdominis muscle. If the tone of the transverse abdominis muscle is good the spine assumes its rigid shape and there is no change in the trunk when one or both feet come up off the floor.

Very often another muscle the rectus abdominis, our sit ups muscle wants to get involved but it has no role to play here. The rectus abdominis draws the pelvis and ribcage closer to one another, but that is not the action in feet three inches off the floor. The trunk wants to be stable, the spine rigid and the transverse abdominis muscle should provide that stability.

Not to be too dramatic but developing tone in the transverse abdominis muscle to accomplish this goal can go a long way towards alleviating back pain in many individuals.

A Tight Psoas and Pinched Sacroiliac Joint

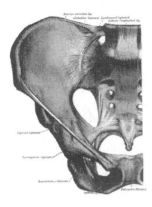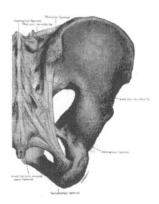

All too many people have a tight psoas muscle if not two tight psoas muscles. The expression of a tight psoas starts with a basic pattern and can go in many directions if left uncared for. Unfortunately any tightening of either psoas muscle is going to affect the alignment and freedom of the sacroiliac joints.

The psoas major attaches to the base of the rib cage (T12) and the lumbar spine (L1-40) before moving forward and down to cross the rim of the pelvis. It then moves backwards to connect to the back half of the inner thighbone, or femur.

The sacroiliac joints are between the sacrum

and the ilium (part of the hip bone) connecting the pelvis together at the back of the body. Nothing in the body works in isolation so any time the psoas becomes misaligned it will affect the sacroiliac joints.

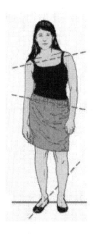

The initial manifestation of a tight psoas usually presents itself in the following way— the tight psoas shortens pulling the femur bone up into the hip socket and pulls the leg, and often the hip forward rotating it externally. This also tends to turn the foot out slightly even elevating the arch of that foot. At the same time the upper portion of a tight psoas both pulls the hip socket up and the shoulder down.

That is the patterns we see in the picture to the left. This primary pattern can morph in different ways depending on how the spine reacts to the torque that arises from a tight psoas and can ultimately affect the opposite shoulder and the ribcage. When both psoas are tight there are a host of other configurations to be found.

But dealing simply with this first pattern that I mentioned, the external rotation of the leg and the hiking of the hip have to adversely affect the sacroiliac joints. The leg comes forward and turns out, rotating the ball of the femur head from the natural place in its socket. That external rotation translates to the hip as well, impinging the sacroiliac joint on that side. Sacroiliac pain is often a result of a tight psoas even though the pain is referred and not felt in the psoas itself.

Everyone is tighter on one side of the body than the other so everyone has a psoas that is tighter as well. If you look in a mirror it is likely that one shoulder is higher or lower than the other. This is one of the first landmarks I look for in a new client. I check the level of the shoulders and then the level and torque of the hips.

But just because one psoas is tighter than the other doesn't necessarily mean that the sacroiliac joint is impinged. There is a degree of a tight psoas that we can all get away with, but if the sacroiliac is suffering, it is likely that a tight psoas is involved in the pain and its ultimate relief.

The Psoas Major and the Urinary Bladder

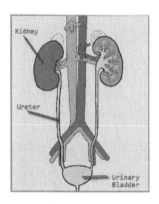

To me there is a relationship between the psoas major and the urinary bladder but I might be making it up though my intuition tells me that it's true. I have been to a number of medical intuitives over the years that I would promptly make fun of for describing themselves that way. Now lo and behold, even though I would never call myself a medical intuitive, intuition truly drives the work I do.

I have had the good fortune to work with a number of doctors with back pain over the years and I have been able to help many of them with my walking program and retraining their basic movement patterns to better serve their spine, pelvis and whatever else was ailing them. My rap is pretty basic—there is a design to the way the body is supposed to work and I try my best to explain in either anatomical or lay terms how that design can help them.

Many years ago after the second or third Psoas Release Party! workshop that I offered (which remains my favorite and most popular offering), I got an email from an attendee who reported that although she didn't come to the workshop for urinary bladder related issues, after an hour and a half of concentrated release work, she slept through the night without getting up to pee four or five times for the first time in a decade.

Obviously this blew my mind at the time because to be honest I was swimming in uncharted territory myself, learning on the fly about this mysterious and profound muscle. It didn't take a big leap in my imagination to think that a short tight psoas could disturb the urinary bladder and create an environment that would make someone pee repeatedly through the night.

So last week when I worked with a doctor who specializes in urinary bladder issues, I went a step too far in saying that a tight psoas could press against the bladder when sleeping to cause someone to urinate multiple times over the course of the night. She looked at me in a not very kind way and said, "Well you just lost me there, because the psoas is about three inches away from the urinary bladder."

I did my best to recover, but thankfully this happened at the tail end of the session, and I was able to slink away to look at my anatomy texts, which along with Google is where I do most of my learning. Sure enough, the urinary bladder and psoas live in different counties, though all anatomy pictures show the same size urinary bladder, which doesn't account for the amount of fluid in them, and long happy psoas muscles.

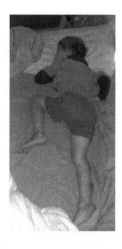

For me, the idea that the psoas and urinary issues are connected is because a tight or traumatized psoas can't sit back into the bowl of the pelvis and ends up closer to the bladder than a happy psoas might. Plus the tight miserable psoas might push the abdominal contents into the urinary bladder. Finally, I think sleep position and the psoas can mess with the urinary bladder depending on how we are situated. I try to get people to avoid hiking one knee higher than the other which I think can affect our need to pee.

I know the doc was right about the literal anatomy of the psoas and urinary bladder but I have seen the effect of release work and sleep position on many clients. I offer my advice and am happy to hear back if it worked—and it doesn't always. I am also happy to be wrong about something because that is often when I do my best learning. And in the eight years since that first woman mentioned an ease in nighttime peeing, I have heard the same thing from many many clients.

Most importantly for the pure joy that I get from what I do, I love that it all remains something of a mystery, like the psoas itself.

Psoas Major Pain and Your Foot

Psoas major pain can be fairly amorphous and problems with the psoas can manifest as lower back pain, hip pain, groin pain, as well as knee, shoulder, neck, and foot pain. Is that enough for you? But foot pain you ask? Really, foot pain? Well, one of my pet phrases is "Your big toe is your psoas".

The psoas major attaches on the back half of the inner thigh and along the entire lumbar (lower) spine as well as the bottom of the middle (thoracic T12) spine. The psoas needs to be aligned on the back half of the inner thigh in order to work its true magic as a muscle that holds the spine successfully on top of the pelvis.

If you are standing on your feet or walking, and grounding effectively through the inside (which doesn't mean collapsing your arch) you will be activating the inner upper thigh, particularly a muscle called adductor magnus which attaches to your sit bone (ischial tuberosity) as well as the pubic bone. When this inner thigh muscle activates it helps to rotate the leg internally which sets the psoas into the back plane of the body so that it can do its thing, and a powerful thing it is.

One of the issues that tends to lead to psoas major pain is that when tight the psoas is pulled into the front plane of the body. When the psoas major is constricted it externally rotates the inner thigh and foot, pulling the thigh forward and open, while hiking up the hip and pulling the shoulder down. This is usually the beginning phase of psoas tightness that can actually get much worse pulling the ribs and spine an all different directions.

Psoas major pain as it relates to the foot or the big toe shows itself because the tightness of the psoas major pulls the foot out of its ability to ground evenly through the big toe. This often shows itself in the affected foot seeming to have a high arch. When a foot is aligned this way it is difficult to ground through the whole foot compounding everything.

This doesn't always show in foot pain—this same alignment can affect and hurt the knee in a similar fashion. It is a big conundrum though because the tight psoas major doesn't allow the foot to ground to set the psoas back at its base and the foot that can't ground through its entirety can't help to activate adductor magnus which supports the psoas.

So what is a body to do to alleviate psoas major pain? Release the psoas out of its tight environment—which doesn't always mean stretching—and change your movement patterns to access the inner foot with each step. Those are two great places to start.

Accommodating the Psoas When Sleeping

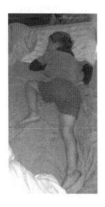

The picture above is my son Reggie. His sleep position mirrors how I slept for the first forty years of my life. One knee hiked up, basically sleeping on the stomach which is just awful for the spine but easy for the psoas muscle. Technically this isn't full on stomach sleeping which is even worse but really, who wants to win a misery contest?

Sleeping on the stomach flattens the curve of the lumbar spine from which no good can come. Sleeping with one knee raised over the other torques the pelvis for the duration of sleeping. Again no good can come from a pelvis that is mis-aligned for hours at a time. Why we do this is another story. I have always felt that the body finds itself in this position as a means of accommodating the psoas that might be tight and which will be much more comfortable with the leg and hip flexed.

For years I woke up with a stiff and achy back, and when I finally committed to sleeping on my side with my legs together and slightly bent, it didn't take long for a lot of my nightly discomfort to pass. Personally, I didn't need to tie my legs together to stop them from separating but I know plenty of people who had to go that far in order to change a lifelong habit.

The classic manifestation of the psoas when tight is for the affected leg and foot to be shortened into the hip socket and turn out with the pelvis and shoulder of the same side to draw closer to each other. The whole affected side shortens. The thing is that I don't think Reggie has a particularly tight psoas so I am not exactly sure why he gravitates towards this position unless the pattern was in my DNA that I shared with him because he has never seen me sleep that way (my daughter never sleeps in this position).

So many people carry around aches and pains that are relatively easy to resolve but require a conscious approach to repetitive actions that we take for granted. Most people do not for a second consider that their sleep position could be harmful. And then there are those who intuited that the way that they sleep could be a problem due to the way they wake up but still don't make the leap to necessary change.

There are injuries that we suffer as a direct result of an action—a car accident, a fall down stairs—but there are also repetitive stress injuries that add up over years of poor patterning. While I realize that most people wouldn't consider sleeping as the cause of a repetitive stress injury I don't see why not.

The Psoas and Iliacus Muscles

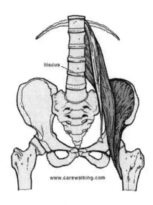

The iliopsoas muscle group is made up of three muscles— psoas major, psoas minor and iliacus. The iliacus starts along the rim of the pelvis lying behind the psoas. The iliacus and psoas then meet to share a common tendon that attaches on the lesser trochanter a small knob of bone on the back half of the inner thigh. This is the only tendon that attaches to this bone in contrast to the greater trochanter on the outer thigh that has many muscles attaching to it including the piriformis which, along with the psoas are the only two muscles in the body that connect the legs to the spine.

When standing the psoas and iliacus lift the leg forward for walking among other things. When lying down the psoas and iliacus can lift the trunk from the floor like a sit up. The iliacus because of its attachment to the pelvis and leg acts only on the hip joint and controls hip movement when involved in twisting the hips for things like kicking.

It is a short and strong muscle creating a good deal of the power required for flexion but like the psoas it is susceptible to becoming short and tight especially due to a sedentary lifestyle. The psoas and iliacus are among the most important muscles in the body but the iliacus is often left out of the discussion when focusing on the all mighty psoas major.

The Psoas Minor Is a Devolving Muscle

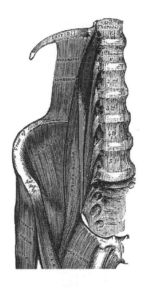

Consult almost any anatomy book and you will read that the psoas minor, one third of the iliopsoas muscle group, is a devolving muscle absent from fifty percent of the population. After reading that in a number of anatomy books it became my standard line when talking about the psoas minor.

The psoas minor attaches to the sides of T12

and L1, the base of the ribcage and top of the lumbar spine, and the disc in between the two vertebrae. It inserts into the pelvis along the pubic ramus into the pectineal line and the iliopectineal eminence which is where the ilium and pubis of the hip bone meet, as well as into the iliac fascia.

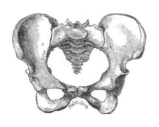
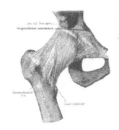

My theory about why it might be a devolving muscle, and this is based purely on conjecture, is that it was replaced by the rectus abdominis in terms of function. In a horse for example the psoas minor functions to flex the spine when still and stabilize the spine in motion. It seems to me that the arch of the lumbar spine created by the psoas major when we came to stand took the psoas minor out of play and the rectus abdominis took over to provide flexion for the spine.

As I mentioned when I first started teaching I

would talk about the psoas minor as a devolving muscle. But then a number of years ago I was attending a workshop offered by Bonnie Bainbridge Cohen, the creator of Body Mind Centering. At some point in the workshop she mentioned that she thought everyone had a psoas minor. She had been working with bodies for years and years and she had always felt the presence of the psoas minor.

After that workshop I was happy to start teaching that everyone has a psoas minor. Why not? Her word is pretty much gospel for me. Fast forward a year or two to another workshop where I was chatting with one of the senior BMC teachers, and as it happens at these events, the psoas minor came up.

I shared with her my change in tone after the prior workshop and she related the same thing with a very interesting twist. In between these two workshops this teacher had gone to a cadaver lab where you get to dissect bodies. Before the work began the BMC teacher mentioned Bonnie's psoas minor thoughts to the leader of the workshop and they went around and checked all the bodies.

Of the thirty-nine bodies in the room only one had a psoas minor. When the BMC teacher related this to Bonnie she was nonplussed and reported, (I paraphrase)" Well, I feel it."

The iliopsoas is a magical muscle.

The Balancing Act of the Psoas and Piriformis Muscles

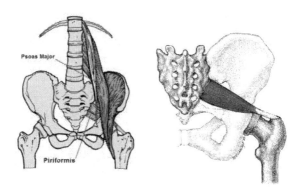

The psoas and piriformis muscles are two muscles that connect the legs to the spine (gluteus maximus is the third). Together—psoas from the front and piriformis in back– they work to keep the spine afloat above the pelvis. The psoas pulls down from the front and the piriformis pulls in the same direction from behind.

When it comes to back pain and dysfunction you can't have trouble in one of these muscles without it affecting the other. When it comes to good posture and spot-on movement patterns the psoas and piriformis muscles are meant to lead the way towards grace and stability.

One way to see this is that the spine is strapped onto the legs at the front and the back by the psoas major and piriformis. If they are both long and toned the spine can sit directly on top of the pelvis. If the psoas major is tight it will pull the lumbar spine forward which will pull the upper spine backwards. Once this happens there is no way for the piriformis to live in its proper place. If the piriformis is tight it pulls the feet wider than parallel and also turns the inner thighs towards the front plane of the body. Once the inner thighs have moved even slightly forward the psoas major loses the tension across the rim of the pelvis that it needs for optimal functioning.

The forward and downward pull of the psoas on the lumbar spine is counteracted by the downward pull of the piriformis on the sacrum. If the pelvis is aligned correctly it is possible for this to happen and these two muscles will help to hold the spine aloft with minimal excess force. Unfortunately I meet few people with a well aligned pelvis and as a result the imbalance of the psoas and piriformis muscles affects all parts of their lives.

The failure of the psoas and piriformis in pulling off their balancing act manifest across the full spectrum of our activities—sitting, standing, walking, running and even sleeping will be influenced by the relationship of the two important muscles.

Three Hip Flexors: Iliopsoas, Sartorius and Rectus Femoris

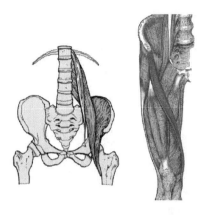

Flexion (drawing the legs towards the trunk or making your bicep pop, for example) is a primary piece of our fear response and human beings are a terrified bunch. This fear manifests in the pelvis through a chronic shortening or engagement of muscles and keeps us stuck in a state of constant alarm. Our body flexes and extends and rotates and we are forever searching for balance in the front, back and sides of the body to allow for these movements to be successful. The search is all too often in vain.

One common place of imbalance is the hip flexors. The hip flexors are the three muscular options for bringing the leg closer to the trunk. With good posture and movement patterns they all work together endlessly in the course of your day.

Sartorius is the longest muscle in the body and I'm sure that I am being naive when I call it fairly inconsequential. It begins on the upper rim of the pelvis crossing the thigh to attach on the inside of the knee. Long and thin it gets a functional assist from the femur bone with which it articulates. In addition to its role as a hip flexor, the sartorius abducts (pulls away) and laterally rotates the hip, and helps with knee flexion. Picking up your foot to look at the bottom of your shoe displays the sartorius in action.

Of the three hip flexors psoas major is the strongest and the only one that connects to the spine. Iliospas is the meeting of the psoas major muscle and the iliacus. The iliacus lines the wall of the pelvis before forming a common tendon with the psoas major to connect at the lesser trochanter, a small bump of bone on the back half of the inner thigh. The psoas major connects along the lower spine. We think the psoas is the most important muscle in the body—it holds us up, walks us through life, and warehouses the trauma we can't deal with in the moment.

Rectus femoris is one of the four quadriceps muscles and though it is a hip flexor, poor postural alignment renders it moot in my book (the same goes for psoas and sartorius for that matter). All four of the quadriceps meet to form the patella tendon, connecting to the shin below the knee. Rectus femoris connects to the pelvis which makes it a hip flexor, while the other three muscles of the quadriceps (the vastus), act to stabilize the knee in extension.

Healing comes with knowledge and the more you know about your body and the way it works, the easier and more likely it will be to change patterns that might have been hindering you your whole life. The hip flexors can hold you back or make your motor hum. Good posture and happy hip flexors allow for a body that welcomes the fear response only to process it and let it go.

The Psoas Major Attaches at the Back of the Body

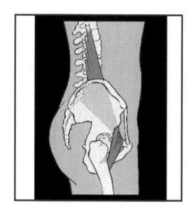

It's all about the psoas. A psoas major muscle in good working order is the engine that drives the body. When we are walking well the psoas initiates movement forward rescuing the body from imminent fall over and over again. A very wise student who also happened to be named Wise made an off-hand comment to me during a yoga class I was teaching many years ago. One day in class I was babbling on, as I do, when she looked at me and said: "You have to realize that the psoas is a back-body muscle."

A few years later, I began to understand what she meant and that awareness is now the cornerstone of what I teach. The psoas major connects at the back of the inner thigh and along the lumbar vertebrae. If the legs are directly under the hips the psoas is pulled into natural tension moving forward from the inner thigh to cross the pelvis and back again to connect to the lower spine. This tension is what creates and maintains the lumbar curve.

It also helps in keeping the spine upright over the pelvis because when the psoas major moves across the pelvis pulling the lumbar vertebrae forward and down, the erector muscles of the spine lengthen up to support the head above the shoulders. This is the pulley action that I have written about before. A pulley is a simple machine that allows the rope that encircles it to generate force. The hip bone is the pulley and the psoas is the rope. This pulley action only happens if the psoas major is situated at the back of the body both above and below the pelvis.

If we tuck the pelvis and allow the thighs to move forward of the hips the psoas is no longer a back-body muscle and we lose all of the good energy that is created by simply aligning the psoas correctly.

Supporting the Psoas Major:
The Holy Trinity of Muscle Groups

Our bones hold us up, and our muscles move us. Our bones are connected by ligaments that are by nature very strong and taut. They don't have much give and they shouldn't change much in tone over the course of a lifetime (with exceptions of pregnancy and other hormonal situations). Muscles are very different. They only have tone if we exercise them to develop their strength and balance. Some people are born stronger than others but everyone needs to do the work to build muscle tone to support the alignment of our bones and allow for the chance of having good posture.

I refer to three muscle groups as the holy trinity, working to support the ideal positioning of my favorite muscle, the psoas major. For the psoas major to be the wonder muscle that it is designed to be, it must be properly situated at its top and bottom, and it can't find that placement by itself.

These three muscle groups are the adductors, muscles of the inner thigh; the levator ani, muscles of the pelvic floor; and the eight abdominal muscles.

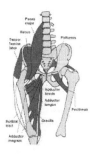

There are five adductors muscles of the inner-thighs. They move the leg in toward the midline and help stabilize the pelvis. The shortest adductor is the pectineus, which attaches high up on the inner thigh and into the pelvis. The longest, gracilis, attaches to the pelvis and all the way down to the shin. And the three middle muscles are adductor magnus, longus and brevis.

All of these muscles attach around the pubic bone. But the adductor magnus, the biggest of them, attaches in two places — the pubic bone and one of your sit bones, the ischeal tuborosity. As a result of this second connection, the adductor magnus is responsible not just for moving your leg to the midline but also assists with internal rotation. And that ability to rotate the leg inward is an absolute key to stabilizing and setting the psoas major.

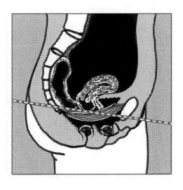

The muscles of the are called the levator ani. Three muscles form a sling at the bottom of the pelvis that connects the tailbone to the pubis. This mass of muscle, about the thickness of your palm, is responsible for holding the pelvic organs in place and for control of rectal and urogenital function. Not only are these muscles bearing a lot of weight from above; they are also pierced by orifices that weaken the pelvic floor merely by their presence.

Continence is high on my list of priorities, and the pelvic floor and continence are dancing partners that we must train and respect. Because these muscles are involved with your eliminative functioning, they have more resting tone than any other muscle in the body and are almost always active—or you'd be peeing all night long. The pelvis and the muscles surrounding it serve a role unique to us bipedal mammals. Just like the psoas major, which is relatively dormant in quadrupeds but wakes up when standing upright brings it into positive tension across the rim of the pelvis, the pelvic floor has a much different role in the biped.

If you think of a dog or a cat or a horse, their pelvis is the back wall of the body rather than the floor. This leaves the organs in a dog to rest on the belly. In standing bipeds, the organs sit right on top of this muscle group, which frankly has enough to do without its newfound responsibility.

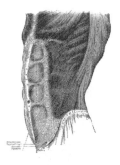

The final group of the holy trinity is the abdominal muscles, equally important for many different reasons. You have eight abdominal muscles—four pairs. All four sets of these muscles move in different directions though they are connected both through tendons and the fascia. The deepest of them is the transverse abdominis. It wraps from the back to the front, meeting at the linea alba a line of connective tissue that runs from the base of the rib cage to the pubic bone. We often refer to the transverse as one muscle, but it is two muscles that meet in the middle. This deep muscle when properly toned, provides a great deal of support for the lumbar spine.

The next layer of abdominal muscles consists of the internal and external obliques, which are angled in opposite directions. These muscles help in twisting, rotating, bending and flexing the trunk and are also active when we exhale.

The third set of abdominal muscles is the rectus abdominis, the "six-pack." This pair of muscles runs vertically, connecting at the pubis at its base and the sternum and three ribs at its top. An anatomical aside about the six-pack: The body has interesting and different ways of compensating for dilemmas of length and space. The length between the pelvis and the rib cage is really too big for one long muscle to provide support. As a result we have tendinous insertions that fall between what are actually ten small muscles. So we really build ten-packs, but we only see six of them. This pack is formed when we make these individual muscles big enough so that they essentially pop out from the tendons that surround them. Muscle is designed to stretch; tendons are not.

The physical and emotional health of the human body depends on the psoas major muscle that is well aligned and properly toned. This only happens if this holy trinity of muscle groups are aligned and toned as well.

Does your Bra Strap Slip? It Might be Your Psoas

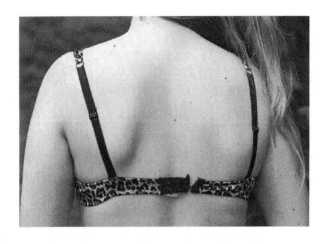

Does your Bra Strap Slip?

Can every issue in life really be related to, or about, the psoas? It's possible. I love my work because I truly never know where it will lead me. I am a de- tective in search of clues that will help people deal with whatever body issues they present to me. And I get presented with some wild stuff. I don't subscribe to any one method though, I think many of them have merit and I am happy to borrow/ steal an idea, or an exercise, that suits my needs.

People need to know how their body works if they want to change the way their body moves and functions. That's the main thread of my approach—if you know how your body is designed to work, you will make better use of the design.

Bras are designed to stay on top of the shoulders. Someone was in the studio the other day and in the course of a session her bra strap slipped a number of times off of the same shoulder. She replaced it unconsciously until I commented on it and she said it happens all the time.

I asked her, as I ask everyone, if she could feel that one shoulder was lower than the other. She replied in the negative but I could see the beginning of a light bulb turning on above her head. She arrived with back pain and didn't expect to be talking about her under garments but…

In fact, the shoulder that the bra strap slipped from was her lower shoulder and also the side of her tight psoas which is what I believe was causing her back pain. Was this the answer to her pain? Of course not; but it was a little kernel of information that could help her get a sense of her body over time.

We did all of the usual things I do in an initial session- worked on standing upright instead of leaning backwards, checked the tone of her core (inner thighs, pelvic floor, and abdominals), and introduced the psoas as the muscle of walking, standing, and trauma.

At the end of the session I told her that she would know if the work that we did together was working if after a good long time she noticed that months had gone by since her bra strap had slipped. That might be an insignificant thing to some, especially men, but could be a truly useful insight for others.

Whatever works is the way I look at it.

Leg Length Discrepancy and a Tight Psoas Major

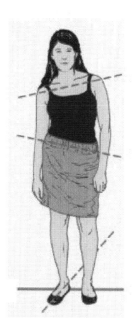

Many people suffer from a leg length discrepancy and this is almost always an issue with the tone of the psoas major rather than with the length of the bones of the skeleton. The body can be divided up in a number of ways—top and bottom, inside and out, back and front, and for today's discussion, left and right. The legs, follow a very cool 1, 2, 3, 4, 5 pattern of bones—one femur for the upper leg; two shin bones; three bones for the ankle; four for the mid-foot; and five toes. The coolest aspect of this pattern is that each bone on the opposite side is exactly the same length and breadth.

In rare cases people are born with bones of different sizes and very often traumatic injuries can affect the length of the bones; but for the most part the hard bits of our skeleton are equal to each other when they exist in pairs. So getting that out of the way leaves us with our psoas major muscle and its ability to wreak havoc on our bodies.

A tight psoas major can take on many patterns. A classic, and I think primary pattern, is when the psoas both pulls the leg up into its hip socket at the bottom and pulls the rib cage down towards the hip at the top. I say primary because I think this is the first tightening pattern for all psoas. In some cases the assorted torque and pull on the spine and ribcage can get much more extreme leading to scoliosis and even a hunchback.

Everyone has a leg length discrepancy—it is merely a matter of degree. If you don't know which one of your legs is shorter than the other here are a few things to look for to figure it out. Very often one foot turns out more than the other—that is your shorter leg. One hip is usually higher than the other- the higher hip is your shorter leg. One shoulder is often lower than the other—that side will be your shorter leg. If you have never observed these details about yourself spend some time looking in the mirror to explore your physical body.

Everyone should get to know themselves, but to use one of my favorite quotes from the German writer Goethe, "Know myself. If I knew myself, I'd run away". And I'll throw in a Ben Franklin quote for good measure. "There are three things extremely hard: steel, a diamond, and to know one's self."

How to work with this discrepancy is another story entirely. One of my favorite psoas releases, Foot on a Block, addresses leg length discrepancy directly. You can do this release on your shorter side, or both sides, feeling what it is like to stand both before and after. It can be a fairly radical feeling even though the exercise only takes about thirty seconds.

There is another very important issue when it comes to leg length discrepancy and yoga practice. The shorter leg is the tighter leg which is not going to have the same range of motion as the looser leg. Many people are right handed and our dominant side is often our shorter side. This is a hypothetical but let's say that your right side is tighter and the ability to stretch it is limited both physically and emotionally. Then you move to work your left side, or more open side, and the available stretch is deeper and feels better—so you dive into it.

Unfortunately, if you can relate to that feeling, you are likely increasing your imbalance and leg length discrepancy with every yoga pose that you do. It is very hard to approach the practice from the point of view of limiting yourself, but everyone should really be stretching to the limit of their tighter side and be focusing on bringing the body into balance rather than just stretching both sides as much as you can.

Psoas Major and Rectus Abdominis

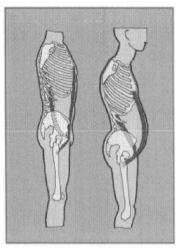

The psoas major muscle and the rectus abdominis muscle have an important relationship inside the body even though they don't literally work together. Muscles relate to each other in many different ways. Sometimes they work in opposition—for the hamstring to lengthen the quadriceps must shorten. This happen through the process of reciprocal inhibition and most often occurs in muscles that live on opposite sides of a bone. Muscles are not elastic and therefore cannot naturally retract after stretching.

Muscles also work synergistically—they help the opposite pairs fulfill their function when needed. The tensor fascia latae synergistically helps the psoas major with hip flexion and internal rotation.

Other muscles work together though they aren't literally connected- the levator ani (pelvic floor) and the diaphragm should do the same thing at the same time to achieve optimal function. Some of these relationships are clear-cut like the hamstring and quadriceps, but other like the psoas major and rectus abdominis are more complicated.

The Psoas Major and the Abdominal Contents

The contents of the trunk, below the ribcage and above the pelvis are suspended within a "box" of muscles. The diaphragm and the levator ani are the top and bottom of the box, and the psoas major and the rectus abdominis at the back and front of the box. The abdominal contents include the intestines, the liver, the bladder and the kidneys. The tone of the muscles that box the organs in can have a major impact on the way the organs function.

I've written before about lower back pain and the rectus abdominus. Sit ups are not the answer for back pain though they are often recommended. Too many sit ups or an overdeveloped rectus abdominis can also be a problem when we have a tight psoas major. A long and happy psoas major muscle lives deep in the bowl of the pelvis creating a sort of shelf alongside the curve of the sacrum. A tight psoas major is pulled forward from the back of the pelvis and basically loses its curve and shelf like qualities.

When this happens the abdominal contents are thrust forward as well and in extreme cases the belly is pushed out. But the belly can only be pushed out if the rectus abdominis is soft enough to allow this forward thrust. If the rectus abdominis is tight from too many sit ups or crunches, it will have no room to accommodate the organs that are being pushed forward.

This environment—tight psoas major and tight rectus abdominis— can have a tremendous effect on digestion, breathing, menstruation and more. If the psoas major and the rectus abdominis have their proper tone the abdominal contents can live happily within the bowl of the pelvis and below the ribcage.

Creating good tone in the abdominal "box" would go a long way towards a finely tuned body but there are many factors working against us. A tight psoas major most often needs to be released rather than stretched and the tone of the rectus abdominis is usually a victim of poor posture and is rarely aligned correctly.

For the psoas major and rectus abdominis to live in harmony we must find our way to better posture and movement patterns. It can't be done without awareness and concentration but that doesn't mean it's not worth the effort.

Is the Psoas Major a Hip Flexor?

Technically the psoas major is not a hip flexor in the traditional sense of flexion. Flexion in the body is when two body parts are brought closer to one another. The psoas major is the most important muscle in the body for a number of reasons.

- It is the muscle most responsible for holding us upright when standing correctly. The psoas major created the lumbar curveof the spine when we came up to stand from all fours- and it is this curve that allows us to be upright with the help of the psoas and other muscles.

- The psoas is the muscle that walks us through life. With every correct step we take the brain tells the psoas to move the leg forward.

- The psoas is the warehouse for the body's fear and trauma. The body is meant to process energetic stimuli both good and bad — and then let go of the nervous energy that is created in the never ending search for balance or homeostasis. When the nervous energy gets stuck in the body it tends to reside in the psoas.

I often refer to the psoas as a hip flexor because of the connection between flexion and our fear response. When we fear we flex; when we fear too much we stay flexed. This condition of staying flexed is what keeps the nervous energy that gets stuck in the body in the psoas.

But technically the psoas shouldn't flex. In a happy and healthy body the psoas should always lengthening. The quadriceps muscle of the leg is a hip flexor. When engaged it extends the knee and draws the thigh closer to the trunk. Many people mistakenly think that their quadriceps muscle is the main muscle for walking but that job falls to the psoas.

The way it works is that rather than flexing the leg forward at the command of the brain the psoas should swing the leg forward. Swinging is much different that flexing. For the psoas to work this way, though, the body must be functioning at a high level with loose joints and long muscles. Very often tightness in the hip joint or the lower back restricts the psoas from swinging, let alone flexing, and then walking leaves the psoas major behind, and the physical action of moving forward is accomplished by compensatory muscles.

The Inner Foot and the Inner Thigh
(and the Psoas Major)

Pressing down on the inner foot activates the muscles of the inner upper thighs. Accessing the deep core of the body, where all the good action is, requires this type of movement through the inner extremities.

The issue is that people tend to bear the body's weight on the outer portions of the body instead of the inner:

- We wear out our shoes on the outside.

- We tend to be very tight in the IT band of the outer hip.

- Watching students in Downward Dog in yoga class, I find that most students bear the weight of the arms in the outer heel of the palm.

Grounding weight on the inside of the foot helps to align and use the psoas major muscle to its mechanical advantage—which requires that the psoas be situated on the back half of the body at its top and bottom. When the psoas lives in the back plane of the body it can be used like a pulley essentially holding the spine up above the pelvis. The outer foot pulls the psoas towards the front plane of the body, tucking the pelvis along the way, while the inner foot allows the inner thighs to tone and move slightly backwards.

It is pretty easy to feel the difference that bearing weight on the inside and outside of the foot makes:

- Come to stand in your natural posture.

- Roll weight to outside of the foot feeling the outer thighs. They should tone when you do that.

- Take your thighs back, untucking the pelvis, and roll to the inside of the foot. The inner thighs should activate more than the outer thighs.

- Weight on the outer foot adds up to a tight IT Band. Weight on the inner foot gives your inner thighs the chance to develop the tone required to align the psoas.

The Psoas Major and Sit Ups

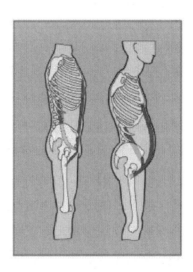

We all need a strong and balanced core. We all want a long and strong psoas major muscle. These two factors are equally important but they often get in each other's way in the search for a functional body.

The trunk is a rectangle split in two—the upper half is the heart and lungs and the lower half is the digestive organs. On the top we have the ribcage encasing these vital organs against damage and on the bottom the intestines, stomach, liver and such live within a box of muscles. The top and bottom of this box is the diaphragm, our main muscle of breathing, and the levator ani, or pelvic floor. These two muscles are actually meant to work together synergistically.

The psoas major makes up the back of the box and the rectus abdominis, our sit ups muscle, is the front of the box. Between these four muscles, the intestinal organs hang in a bag from the spine. These organs need room to move and the freedom to do their jobs. If the space in the box that they live in becomes constricted, they will not be able to work effectively, and digestion, among other functions, is impacted (pun intended).

We all need to do sit ups, even though I often say that sit ups are bad for you. I don't mind being a walking contradiction in this case because both of those statements are true. My basic take on the body is that we are all splayed open long in the front and short in the back. If this is true we need to bring the front of the body into balance with the back of the body, which will require shortening the rectus abdominis as its length determines the space between tween the pelvis and the rib cage.

I mentioned earlier about the relationship between the transverse abdominis and the rectus abdominis and the need to have tone in the transverse abdominis before doing work on the rectus abdominis. There is a different concern when it comes to the psoas major. In an ideal world the psoas major lengthens down the bowl of the pelvis, and the rectus abdominis runs directly down in a straight line from the rib cage to the pubic bone.

If that is the case and there is good tone in the transverse abdominis there is no reason not to work on your sit ups to try and bring balance to the front and the back of the body. But what if the psoas is tight? I often use the example of someone who appears to be skinny with little body fat, yet there is a pot belly sticking out above the waist. To me this is an indication of a tight psoas major that is pulled forward from the back of the pelvis, because when the tight psoas is pulled towards the front of the body the organs don't have anywhere to go but forward and the rectus abdominis goes with it- hence the pot belly.

The problem is that many people, for many

reasons, think that building your core is the anti-dote to back pain. And while it is true— if your psoas is tight and you do a lot of sit ups, shortening the distance between the pelvis and the ribcage, you are effectively limiting the amount of room in the box of organs. The tight psoas pushes the organs forward and the tight rectus abdominis pushes them backwards and no good can come of that. Someone in this position will likely have a hard rather than soft belly due to the pressure on the abdomen.

The order of business should be—release your psoas, tone your transverse abdominis, and then work the rectus abdominis to the length you desire. It always comes back to the consciousness we need to bring to building our bodies. Many things that are important for our bodies require understanding what is going on with underlying structures within. This kind of work takes time and patience but I think it is well worth it.

The Psoas Major Muscle and Lower Back Pain

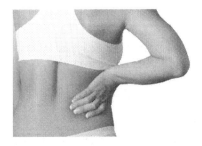

Pain that manifests as a result of psoas major muscle dysfunction can take all forms. We will start by looking at lower back pain. The lower back or lumbar spine is five bones that make up the portion of the spinal column between the pelvis and the rib cage. Whereas the pelvis and ribcage have a bony presence from one side of the body to the other—in between these two structures, there are five bones, the largest five bones of the spine, living directly in the center of the body. These five bones, whose tiny inward curve determines our ability to be upright suc- cessfully, require a great deal of muscle tone to live in the proper alignment.

The psoas major muscle pulls the bones of the lumbar spine forward when it engages or short- ens. If you sit down into a chair, as soon as you stick your butt out and send the thighs backwards towards the seat the psoas moves backwards at its base (the inner thigh) and draws forward and down at its top pulling the lower back forward with it. Hopefully, this is fairly easy to feel.

With this action there is meant to be an opposite reaction. When the psoas major muscle pulls the lumbar vertebrae forward the muscles of the spine— the erector spinea, the multifidus— are all supposed to lengthen up the back, extending the spine, against the downward pull of the psoas major. This is a concept called reciprocal inhibition.

Ideally the psoas works like a pulley system in the body helping to hoist the spine up on top of the pelvis but when this doesn't happen as planned — which is often—due to poor posture and chronically tight muscles, the psoas pulls the lumbar vertebrae forward but the spinal extensors can't provide the opposite lift up. As a result the bones of the lower back compress causing lower back pain in the center of the spine.

There is good pain and there is bad pain. Pain in the joints is almost always bad pain, especially in the joints of the lumbar spine. Dysfunction in the psoas major muscle can manifest in many different forms of pain but this particular lower back pain that is felt in the joints of the lumbar spine requires a lot of skeletal and muscular realignment.

The Psoas Major and Groin Pain:

The Inguinal Ligament

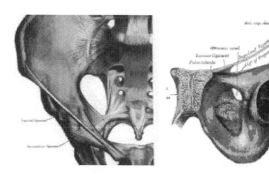

Groin pain can be directly related to the psoas major through the inguinal ligament. Clients come to me with all manners of pain. Back pain, hip pain, knee pain, shoulder pain, and groin pain. To be hyperbolic, which is my favorite way to be, I always say- It's your psoas. I am only half joking. An unhappy psoas major prevents the rest of the body from being content.

There is plenty of knee pain that is directly related to the knee as well as back pain limited to a disc in the spine but there are certain common pains that I find to be associated with the psoas major though the pain radiates from a different part of the anatomy.

The inguinal ligament connects from the anterior superior iliac spine (ASIS) of the ilium to the pubic tubercle of the pubic bone. It passes right above the psoas major essentially strapping it into place. Interestingly, the function of a ligament is to connect one bone to another bone. As you see in the pictures above, the inguinal ligament is connecting to the same bone. To digress a bit, when you are born, the ilium, the pubis, and the ischium are separate bones that fuse over time. So, technically, the argument can be made that the ligament is connecting two separate bones that have simply fused into one.

Back to the psoas major and groin pain. As I said, the inguinal ligament basically runs over the psoas strapping it across the rim of the pelvis. One of the common pains that I mentioned earlier was a wrapping pain that tends to run from the pubic bone up and around the groin to the hip and the lower back. Over time I have come to think that this wrapping pain is a tight psoas major pushing on the inguinal ligament causing the discomfort.

Is One Leg Shorter Than the Other?
Ask the Psoas.

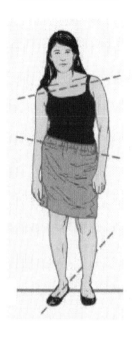

There is no true symmetry across the two sides of the human body. No one is fully ambidextrous. Our skeletal structure is the same on both sides of the body with the corresponding bones all being the same size and shape.

One in a million people might have one leg shorter than the other due to one of the bones being shorter on one side but it is very rare. The reason for our imbalance is that we have a very different musculature on both sides of the body which leads us to having a dominant side. In the same way that everyone is handed, right or left, everyone to one degree or another has one leg shorter than the other.

A few years ago when I went to the Bodies Exhibit here in NYC's South Street Seaport, the aspect of the show that struck me most was viewing the same muscle on both sides of the body. Very often you would have a strong solid muscle on the right side that looks like it was straight out of an anatomy book, and then on the other side there would be this limp and flaccid excuse for a muscle that barely existed.

One leg is shorter than the other most often because of the tightness of the psoas major. Everyone's side to side imbalance varies for different reasons but my take is that leg length discrepancy is mainly due to the psoas muscle and its imbalance. The psoas connects at the base of the rib cage, all along the lumbar spine and then down and back to the back half of the femur, or leg, bone.

When the psoas is tight it pulls the affected leg up into the hip socket and often pulls the hip up towards the rib cage and the rib cage down towards the hip. That is just one of the ways a tight psoas can manifest. But the shortening or pulling up of the leg into the hip socket is usually the first response to any tightening in the psoas muscles.

Walking and Breathing: the Psoas Muscle and the Diaphragm.

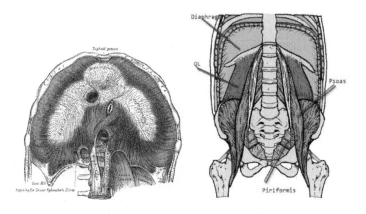

    Walking and breathing are intimately connected through the psoas muscle and thediaphragm muscle. The psoas major is the main muscle of walking, an action ideally initiated deep in the core of the trunk. The psoas connects the spine to the legs attaching on the lower spine (T12, L1-4), before crossing the rim of the pelvis to attach on the back half of the inner thigh. The psoas muscle, if properly aligned is capable of supporting and moving us through space. Its downward pull on the front of the lower spine allows many muscles at the back of the body to lengthen and tone upwards providing support for the head at the top of the spine. When walking it is the work of the two psoas muscles moving in opposition that stimulates a natural and healthy rotation in the pelvis and throughout the spine. Most people use their big thigh muscles (quadriceps) to pull them through life, but if everything works according to design, the psoas is generating our movement and many overworked muscles get to relax.

The diaphragm muscle, a dome shaped muscle at the base of the ribcage, is the essential muscle of breathing. When we inhale the diaphragm is meant to descend allowing air to be drawn into the expanding lungs. At the base of the pelvis, three layers of muscle support the weight of the organs. These pelvic muscles and the diaphragm work synergistically connecting walking and breathing with every successful step. With each inhalation the diaphragm and pelvic floor should lower and with each exhale they should rise back up moving the contents of the trunk with them. Add to this up and down movement the rotational possibilities of the psoas when walking, and every breath and every step we take can tone and massage the entire contents of the trunk..

There are also relationships between the psoas muscle and the diaphragm muscle that literally connect the acts of walking and breathing. There are two tendons for the diaphragm called the crura that extend down and connect to the spine right alongside the psoas attachment. One of the ligaments of the diaphragm (medial arcuate) wraps around the top of the psoas. Finally the diaphragm and the psoas connect through fascia, the webbing that encases the body in both safe and sorry ways. There is a particular fascial grouping that joins the diaphragm, psoas and other hip muscles.

The relationship between these two titans of walking and breathing cannot be understated. Health in one can and will encourage health in the other.

Neighbors: Psoas Major and Quadratus Lumborum

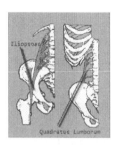

The psoas major and the quadratus lumborum are next door neighbors and you know how it can be if two neighbors don't get along. In fact, to continue the image, they share a driveway which as you might imagine can really complicate things. The psoas major is our favorite muscle and we consider it to be the most important muscle in the body. It is the engine of walking and a warehouse for trauma which makes it very important indeed. Its next door neighbor, the quadratus lumborum ,has a much different nature. It bends the body sideways and back up towards the mid line, and while important, doesn't carry the same weight as the psoas major.

But, as is the case with the psoas' sister muscle, the piriformis, you can't have problems in one without have problems with the other. The psoas major attaches at six points. It inserts on the back half of the inner thigh at its base and then moves forward to cross the rim of the pelvis before moving back towards the spine and up. It connects on all of the vertebrae of the lower spine (lumbar) as well as the bottom vertebrae of the middle spine (thoracic). It connects on each of these vertebrae on the front of the body as well as the costal processes. The costal processes are the little jutting bones on the side of the vertebrae that you can see in the picture above (The psoas major doesn't attach on the costal process of the bottom thoracic vertebrae, only on the body).

The quadratus lumborum originates on the top of the pelvis and connects the pelvis to the rib cage with its attachment on the top ridge. In between, it attaches on the same costal processes as the psoas major. So while these two muscles have completely different functions their mutual connections (the driveway they share) marry them for life.

It is our belief that though the psoas major is the body's most important muscle, there are a host of other muscles that are profoundly affected by its troubles, and quadratus lumborum, along with piriformis, are the two most important muscles that are affected.

It is a chicken and egg equation, but let's say that the psoas major is tight, pulling the lumbar spine forward into an excessive curve. That forward pull takes the quadratus lumborum with it and it will no longer be able to function optimally. When we are teaching people to stand and walk correctly we focus a lot of our attention on the psoas major, but in almost every case, the quadratus lumborum is habitually and chronically tight and fights hard to maintain its long held position. And its long held position is the problem that is pulling the guy in the picture below into his problematic leaning back posture. We think this is due in large part to an underused psoas major and a chronically tight quadratus lumborum.

Psoas Stretch vs Psoas Release?

Psoas stretches are at the foundation of any yoga class even if the teachers and students don't realize it.

As a yoga teacher, it is my job to stretch people, but it wasn't long before I began to come across people who didn't seem to be served by stretching. They would come to class regularly, but their hips or hamstrings or whatever they hoped to lengthen never seemed to give in.

I came to realize that a muscle that is full of tension cannot be stretched free of that tension. In certain cases we must learn to release the tension and/or trauma from a muscle in order to get to the point where we can stretch it.

In the case of the psoas my take is pretty simple; if you have no pain in the lower back, hips, or groin, you should do psoas stretches to your heart's content. While psoas releases would be great for you too, I can see why there wouldn't be a great incentive to lay around for 45 minutes doing as little as possible.

If you are in pain, suffering from tight hips,

lower back pain, groin pain, etc., then psoas release work is a great option. Always with the idea that when you are ready, you get back to deeper psoas stretches.

There are a number of psoas release videos on my blog, my favorite being Constructive Rest Position. They are as much about exploring your psoas and your pelvis as they are about healing. Healing begins with awareness. Psoas releases are about stepping back a little to listen to your body and come to a better understanding of how your body works.

Physical, emotional, and postural health are predicated on a body having loose supple joints with toned muscles. Sometimes a psoas stretch is exactly what you need to accomplish that, but psoas release work is a beautiful way to heal the body and/or compliment a rigorous training program.

The Psoas and Flexion

The Psoas is the body's main hip flexor which is why it is the main muscle of walking, but it plays a deeper maybe more important role as a flexor. Flexors are muscles that bring one body part closer to another one. Flexion's relationship to the nervous system is through our fear response. Our sympathetic nervous system, the system of excitation, from which stems our flight or fight response, manifests through flexion; like all animals in the wild when startled or afraid, we automatically react. The psoas is involved in each of these reactions.

Life is traumatic and this is not necessarily a bad thing. From the big trauma of being born and taking our first breath to the lesser traumas of day-to-day life, we are here to be traumatized and to one degree or another develop an inner support system to heal. Like the pulsing of the heart and the ebb and flow of the tides, the body's trauma/healing interplay is as natural as breathing. When the nervous system doesn't successfully integrate a traumatic event it becomes trapped in the body, very often manifesting through pain and injury to the psoas.

When the processing of trauma doesn't proceed successfully we can get stuck in the sympathetic nervous system. This affects many functions of the body, specifically the psoas and also our breathing. The psoas is intimately connected to our diaphragm, the main muscle of breathing. Both the psoas and the breath can lose the ability to work in an optimal way, and as a result many of our essential functions can become disrupted. The synergistic relationship of the diaphragm and the psoas provide tone and stimulation to many of our organs and when they are not working in harmony the opportunity for dysfunction is increased exponentially.

Physical troubles are the obvious result of problems with the psoas but being stuck in the sympathetic nervous system can cause wide ranging and more troubling emotional effects as well.

Walking, the Psoas and the Diaphragm

According to the body's design, every breath we take should tone and massage the contents of the trunk between the base of the ribs and the base of the pelvis. The diaphragm, a dome shaped muscle at the bottom of the ribcage, is the essential muscle of breathing. At the base of the pelvis a group of muscles called the levator ani support the weight of the organs and help control elimination. The psoas muscle originates on the bottom vertebrae of the thoracic spine and on the top four vertebrae of the lumbar spine. It moves down across the front rim of the pelvis and then moves backwards to insert onto the back half of the inner thigh. As one of the body's main flexors and one of only two muscles that connect the lower and upper body the psoas is largely responsible for walking. The rectus abdominus, otherwise known as the six-pack, runs from the front of the pelvis to the rib cage and sternum directly across from the psoas. These four sets of muscles essentially house the contents of the abdomen. Their placement and tone goes a long way to determining the efficacy of many of our essential functions.

We find an endless array of reciprocal relationships in the body. The pelvic floor and the diaphragm have one of these relationships. In good posture these two structures are level and this is important because they work synergistically. With each inhalation, the diaphragm and pelvic floor should lower fractionally and with each exhale they should rise back up. That top and bottom balance is countered by a front and back dynamic that exists between the psoas and the rectus abdominus. In this relationship with every inhale the psoas settles backwards into the bowl of the pelvis, and the rectus abdominus moves forward allowing for the abdominal contents to be pressed down by the diaphragm. Exhaling brings everything back to the beginning. As you will see below based on the placement of our organs when these structures all move well we are creating the ultimate environment for health.

If everything moves as designed, every breath we take tones, massages and stimulates everything between the diaphragm and the base of the pelvis. Your kidneys live on either side of the psoas. The abdominal aorta moves through the diaphragm and splits into two arteries that follow the path of the psoas into the leg. The bladder and reproductive organs sit in front of the psoas and the stomach and intestines plug into the middle of all this. The large intestine wraps around the small intestine, under the diaphragm and in front of the psoas along the path of the side of the body.

With every step you take a whole host of muscles spring into action. The psoas is drawn down and back through the inner thigh as that leg extends backwards pulling the pelvis back and the lumbar spine is pulled forward. Your rectus abdominus counters that for tone while other abdominal muscles get involved to aid in the natural rotation that moves naturally up through the spine. As you switch legs, the same thing happens on the other side of the body creating a continual rotation through the spine initiated by the psoas. Imagine a washing machine and how it wrings dirt out of your clothes as it works through the wash cycle. When the legs, pelvis, and spine move in harmony with your core muscles, this same action is created in your trunk. The organs all move; toxins get worked out, and healthy tone settles in to organs that are never stagnant.

Finding a healthy walking and breathing pattern involves all of these structures and creates a profoundly healthy and supportive environment for the body.

The Psoas Knows

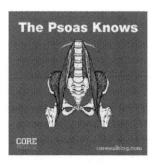

The psoas knows everything that has ever happened in your life. The psoas majoris is an incredible muscle, and certain things that happen in the course of your life, stay locked inside the psoas. It is as if a muscle deep inside your body is making decisions about what your emotional brain can handle. How crazy is that?

Constructive rest position (CRP), a pose that I recommend everyone become friends with, has probably been the single most humbling "thing" I have come across in my life. In constructive rest position a person lies on the floor with the knees bent and the feet flat to the floor. That's it. And then, depending on what your psoas has chosen to hold within its bounds, the magic happens. Or not.

The magic, for what it's worth, takes all forms. A short list of happenings that I have witnessed in CRP include—knees falling involuntarily from side to side, feet slapping the ground, minor convulsions that look like electric shocks, and major convulsions where the body rides waves of movement from within.

My simple take is that the human animal, with its ability to reason, has thwarted the natural mammalian process of excitation followed by relaxation, otherwise known as homeostasis. Animals that can't think the way we do process trauma in a purely instinctual way. They experience it, and let it go, with different animals having different techniques for this type of release. Human beings are different. Some of us process instinctually and don't hold onto the experiences we go through– imagine a soldier in combat who doesn't get post-traumatic stress disorder (PTSD).

Watching someone go through the effects of constructive rest position can be very powerful. And to repeat myself—it is very beautifully humbling. One amazing thing that I have found is that the body doesn't let go in constructive rest until it is ready to, crazy as that might sound.

A while back I had a client who was experiencing extreme reactions in constructive rest and was being woken up in the middle of the night by what she described as electrical charges below her sternum. The coolest thing was, though she was fairly freaked out and wanted to know what was going, she had a smile on her face.

I explained to her that I thought her body wouldn't be taking her on this journey if she wasn't prepared for it. For whatever reason, whatever it was that was coming out of her body had chosen to stay inside up until now. If she wasn't ready to let it out it would continue to stay inside.

It? It? It? What the hell am I talking about "it" that is coming out. Is it trauma, memory, feeling, pain? I don't know but the psoas knows.

A Filet Mignon is the Psoas Major

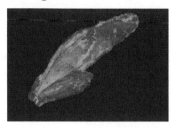

The filet mignon, or tenderloin, that we eat is the psoas major muscle of, in most cases, a cow. The psoas of a cow is very different from the human psoas. In four-legged animals the psoas doesn't touch the pelvis in its journey from the leg to the spine, while the human psoas created the all important lumbar curve of our lower back when it crossed the rim of the pelvis as we came up to stand.

The tenderloin gets its name and subsequent quality for an interesting reason. Not to offend vegetarians, but if you can, put in your mind's eye a butcher's case and see a rib eye or strip steak. These sumptuous cuts get their flavor from the fat marbled within them. But if you can also see a filet mignon, you will notice that it doesn't have fat running through it— it is prized for its fat-less tenderness.

There is an important lesson here to help us understand the psoas. Fat is flavor, but it is also protection and the fact that the psoas has less fat running through and around it means that it is a more vulnerable muscle than most.

I refer to the psoas as the most important muscle in the body for three reasons:

- It is the muscle that holds us up.

- It is the muscle that walks us forward

- It is the muscle that stores all of our unreleased trauma

The third claim is an esoteric reach but I am happy to make it. The psoas is a deep core muscle that can affect the body in profound ways. I don't know what its lack of fat has to do with being our warehouse for trauma, but I would not be surprised if there was a connection. Anyone with thoughts on the matter is invited to please weigh in.

What is the Psoas Muscle?

The psoas is my favorite muscle and also the body's most important muscles for many reasons:

- It is the posture muscle. The awakening of the psoas muscle as we came up to stand created the curve of our lower back that allows us to be upright.

- It is the standing muscle. Along with the piriformis the psoas connects the legs to the trunk and together they hold the spine up on top of the pelvis.

- It is the walking muscle. A body working correctly catches itself falling forward through space with each initiation of the psoas muscle.

- It is the trauma muscle. This means different things for different people. Every body processes stress differently but for everyone the psoas is the main storage unit for the body's response to stimulus. If we don't successfully process and release our stress it will remain in the body and can have debilitating effects on daily functioning both physically and emotionally.

- It is the pain muscle. From my prospective almost all back pain stems from the function/dysfunction of the psoas muscle and the piriformis .

So, what is the psoas muscle? It is the most important muscle in the body that most people have never heard of. However, slowly but surely it is making its way into people's understanding of the body and pain. Learning about the function and use of the psoas muscles can only help us stay healthy and live longer with more vitality.

The Psoas Major in Handstands

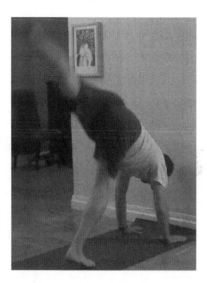

You won't be surprised to read that from my perspective, the psoas major is intimately involved with successful handstands. When working well, the psoas major acts as a pulley system to help extend the spine to its full length— facilitating the erector muscles of the spine and aligning the head, neck and shoulders.

There are many ways to get up into handstands. Gymnasts tend to approach handstands from a standing position, while in yoga we tend to be grounded and go up from downward dog—or for advanced practitioners from uttanasana, standing forward bend. We will look at kicking up into a handstand from downward dog.

Two prevalent tendencies limit people in their attempts to achieve handstands:

- The lifting leg and hip turn out and up when kicking up.
- The spine loses stability and arches too much.

A psoas major that works well creates a certain amount of tension as it crosses the rim of the pelvis. The psoas major attaches on the back half of the inner thigh, moves forward across the rim of the pelvis and goes back again to connect to the lower spine. This back, front, back setup is an important factor in the psoas majors' ability to help the spine stay upright, as well as to get the spine over the arms into a handstand.

Developing movement that emanates from the core is the point of the practice. Engagement and employment of the psoas is the ultimate core connection—it is hard to achieve the stability we seek without getting in touch with our center.

To get up into a handstand, the leg that kicks should stay in the same plane as the trunk and hip. I actually pigeon toe the lifted leg a little to help this process. If my lifting leg stays lined up, the tension/pulley action brought to the psoas as I kick lengthens the spine with reciprocal inhibition making it easier to maintain a solid trunk and to lever the hips over the shoulders.

If my leg doesn't stay in line as I kick, the hip and leg tend to turn open sideways. As soon as this happens, all the tension that my psoas major brought to bear across the pelvis disappears. When this happens the spinal erectors that were extending the back of the spine lose their tone, and with the resulting loss of tone, the hips often move faster than the shoulders and the lower back arches excessively due to the loss of reciprocal inhibition that the engagement of the psoas major created.

A solid trunk and well aligned leg go together in cultivating successful handstands.

The Psoas Major and Back Bending

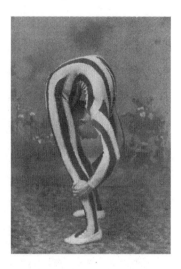

By now, you know that I think the psoas major muscle is the key to healthy walking and standing. This extraordinary muscle is also essential to back bending in yoga. There are only three muscles that connect the arms and legs to the spine. The psoas major and piriformis connect the legs, and the latissimus dorsi connects the arms to the spine and pelvis.

A successful backbend involves an extension of the spine that can't happen without the help of the psoas major and the latissimus dorsi. The psoas must en- gage for the spine to lengthen at the back. This is a result of reciprocal inhibition, one of the body's best magic tricks. For one muscle to lengthen, an- other muscle must shorten. For the muscles of the back and spine (erector spinea among others) to lengthen, the psoas must shorten or engage so that reciprocal inhibition can kick in.

The psoas is the most important muscle in the body and its importance is never more evident than when backbending.

The feet, knees and legs all need to be in the right place for the psoas to do its thing. And its thing in back- bending is to pull forward and slightly down drawing the lumbar vertebrae for- ward. This is the action that allows the opposite lengthening of the erector muscles of the spine.

In order for the psoas to accomplish this it must be correctly aligned at the back half of the inner thigh. The psoas attaches on the lesser tro- chanter, a knob on the back half of the thigh bone. It needs to be in the back of the body in order to create the necessary tension as the muscle crosses the pelvis to attach to the lumbar spine. If it is in the back plane of the body the proper tension is available. This can happen if the feet are grounded and the legs aligned.

The unfortunate tendency is for the feet to roll out and the knees to move out to the side. When this happens, the back half of the inner thigh moves towards the front half of the body and the requisite tension can't manifest. We need the psoas to be properly aligned and engaged for a backbend to successfully lengthen the spine. If this doesn't happen the back is much more likely to bend instead of lengthen, leading to a compression in the bones of the lower spine. I really believe that a majority of students are compressing rather than lengthening the spine.

The psoas is the most important muscle in the body and its importance is never more evident than when backbending.

Psoas Major

The psoas major is the most important muscle in the body. It is both the main muscle of walking and the main muscle of trauma. Here we'll talk about walking. The psoas major, the piri- formis, and gluteus maximus are the only three muscles connecting the upper and lower body. In large part, the balance of the psoas and piriformis muscles is holding the spine upright on top of the pelvis.

Every step you take should be the simple act of the upper body falling forward through space and the nervous system telling the psoas major to pull a leg forward, in order to catch you time and time again throughout the day. Most people are probably taking 5,000 steps a day without thinking about any of them.

Walking is falling and catching yourself over and over and your psoas major should initiate the action of the leg moving forward with the help of a whole host of other muscles. The unfortunate reality is that most people are using the quadriceps, the big muscle of the thigh, to walk when it really is the job of the psoas major.

If you are walking/falling forward through space your legs fall underneath your pelvis and your quadriceps works way less. The quad does its little bit to help but its main responsibility lies elsewhere at the knee. If you fall forward your psoas major begins to take over the action of walking and the body begins to work more in line with its design.

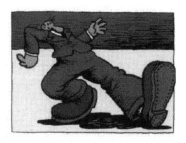

All quads, no psoas major.

The sad part is if you are not falling for- ward through space with the help of the psoas major, you are leaning backwards through space, using way more muscles than you need to be us- ing, employing none of the body's design. Walk- ing is a very simple act when accomplished by the psoas major. When you lean backwards through life you make walking way more difficult than it needs to be.

ACKNOWLEDGEMENTS

I have learned from so many people both in person and in print. Here is a short list of those who influenced this book:

Ida Rolf	Irene Dowd
Therese Bertherat	Liz Koch
John Friend	Bessel van der Kolk
Jenny Otto	Peter Levine
Sandra Jamrog	Tom Myers
Bonnie Bainbridge Cohen	

Many thanks to all of the students who have been patient with me on my path of learning; you have been my true teachers and my true guides.

Thanks as well to artists and models:

Chris Marx, Ida FitzGordon, Christopher Moore, Frank Morris, Jesse Kaminash, Mark Chamberlain, Heather Greer, Molly Fitzsimons, Caitlin FitzGordon

ART CREDITS

Illustrations

Frank Morris: Cover, inside cover, pps 2, 8, 22, 26, 27, 31, 42

Grays Anatomy: pps 5, 10, 17, 18, 30, 35, 36

Beth O'hara: pps vi, 5, 210

Robert Crumb: pps 112, 272

Kevjonesin: p 197

Olek Remesz "Musculi coli base": p 134

Mark Chamberlain: p 137

Video Captures

Heather Greer: pps 57, 59, 60, 62-64, 68, 70-72, 75, 77

Photographs

Molly FitzSimons: pps 65-67, 73, 78-80, 82